P9-EJI-932

www.wadsworth.com

wadsworth.com is the World Wide Web site for Wadsworth and is your direct source to dozens of online resources.

At *wadsworth.com* you can find out about supplements, demonstration software, and student resources. You can also send email to many of our authors and preview new publications and exciting new technologies.

wadsworth.com
Changing the way the world learns®

OKANAGAN UNIVERSITY COLLEGE
LIBRARY
BRITISH COLUMBIA

CLINICAL PRACTICE
WITH ADOLESCENTS

DAVID G. MARTIN
University of Manitoba

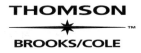

THOMSON

BROOKS/COLE

Australia • Canada • Mexico • Singapore
Spain • United Kingdom • United States

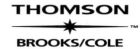

THOMSON

BROOKS/COLE

Executive Editor: Lisa Gebo
Acquisitions Editor: Julie Martinez
Assistant Editor: Shelley Gesicki
Editorial Assistant: Mike Taylor
Technology Project Manager: Barry Connolly
Marketing Manager: Caroline Concilla
Marketing Assistant: Mary Ho
Advertising Project Manager: Tami Strang
Project Manager, Editorial Production:
   Stephanie Zunich

Print/Media Buyer: Nancy Panziera
Permissions Editor: Sue Ewing
Production Service: Andy Sieverman,
   G&S Typesetters
Text Designer: Jeanne Calabrese
Copy Editor: Mimi Braverman
Cover Designer: Denise Davidson
Cover Images: PhotoDisk
Compositor: G&S Typesetters
Printer: Webcom Limited

COPYRIGHT © 2003 Brooks/Cole, a division
of Thomson Learning, Inc. Thomson Learning™
is a trademark used herein under license.

ALL RIGHTS RESERVED. No part of this work covered
by the copyright hereon may be reproduced or used
in any form or by any means—graphic, electronic, or
mechanical, including but not limited to photocopying,
recording, taping, Web distribution, information networks, or information storage and retrieval systems—
without the written permission of the publisher.

Printed in Canada
1 2 3 4 5 6 7 06 05 04 03 02

For more information about our products, contact us at:
Thomson Learning Academic Resource Center
1-800-423-0563

For permission to use material from this text,
contact us by:
Phone: 1-800-730-2214
Fax: 1-800-730-2215
Web: http://www.thomsonrights.com

Library of Congress Control Number: 2002104363

ISBN 0-534-52382-X

Brooks/Cole—Thomson Learning
511 Forest Lodge Road
Pacific Grove, CA 93950
USA

Asia
Thomson Learning
5 Shenton Way #01-01
UIC Building
Singapore 068808

Australia
Nelson Thomson Learning
102 Dodds Street
South Melbourne, Victoria 3205
Australia

Canada
Nelson Thomson Learning
1120 Birchmount Road
Toronto, Ontario M1K 5G4
Canada

Europe/Middle East/Africa
Thomson Learning
High Holborn House
50/51 Bedford Row
London WC1R 4LR
United Kingdom

Latin America
Thomson Learning
Seneca, 53
Colonia Polanco
11560 Mexico D.F.
Mexico

Spain
Paraninfo Thomson Learning
Calle/Magallanes, 25
28015 Madrid, Spain

To the most wonderful grandchildren in the world:
Abigail, Courtney, Ryan, Ian, Susan, and Hayley

CONTENTS

PREFACE

The primary purpose of *Clinical Practice with Adolescents* is to guide and influence the clinical treatment of adolescents by practitioners in a wide range of professions—clinical psychology, counseling psychology, mental health work, occupational therapy, psychiatry, psychiatric nursing, school psychology, social work, and treatment work. The book draws on extensive research literature, but it is designed to be practical and immediately useful to the practitioner. Both coverage and style are intended to be personal and applied.

Because this book is intended to guide practitioners with adolescents, coverage is highly selective and covers several areas. The principle that guides this selectivity is, What information does the practitioner need to work with adolescents in an applied setting? Chapter 1 discusses the rewards and difficulties of working with adolescents and the primary developmental issues adolescents face. Chapters 2, 3, and 4 describe the practical realities of working with individual adolescents. Chapter 2 focuses on ways to establish a therapeutic alliance with an adolescent client. The overall theme of this book is that research evidence tells us that clinical work with adolescents has mostly to do with relationships. Techniques are important, but they are secondary to relationship issues, and different techniques can lead to similarly successful outcomes. The practitioner needs to be familiar with but not constrained by a wide range of methods. Chapters 3 and 4, therefore, present a wide range of techniques, special problems, and intervention methods, especially behavioral and cognitive behavioral methods.

Chapters 5 and 6 give advice about working with groups of adolescents and their families. Group therapy (chapter 5) is presented as a useful approach with adolescents and in the context of demands for cost-effective treatments. Family therapy (chapter 6) is discussed both as a primary format for treatment and as an adjunct to other forms of treatment.

Chapter 7 discusses treatment issues that are unique to particular disorders. As in the rest of the book, this is a highly selective presentation of information that practitioners most often find useful in working with adolescent clients. I make some comments on the process of assessment and diagnosis, but this book is not a guide to assessment or a textbook on abnormal psychology. The emphasis is on practical advice for identifying disorders and on special considerations for treatment.

As mentioned earlier, the guiding philosophy of this book is that the foundation of clinical work with adolescents is the quality of the relationship between the clinician and the adolescent. The practicing clinician needs to know much about technique and theory, but this material is presented in the context of the clinical relationship. This guiding philosophy is frequently supported with citations of research literature throughout the book. In addition, the book includes case examples to illustrate specific points. The most common form that this takes is brief descriptions of scenarios followed by suggestions for what a practicing clinician might say in the situation.

This book is intended for a wide range of professions—clinical psychology, counseling psychology, mental health work, occupational therapy, psychiatry, psychiatric nursing, school psychology, social work, and treatment work—each of which could use it in one or more courses. As a supplemental text, this book could be adopted for a wider range of courses, and it could also be used in clinical practica and field placements in several professions. Some of the workers in these professions will have been trained in formal university degree programs, and some will have been trained in certificate programs in community colleges. The title, *Clinical Practice with Adolescents*, is designed to be broad enough to appeal to virtually all workers in the human services professions who deal with adolescents. Unless I am discussing a specific profession, I use the terms "clinician" and "practitioner" to include many professionals as readers.

The potential students to whom this book will appeal range from advanced undergraduates in university, college, or community college programs to graduate students in programs with an emphasis on clinical work with adolescents. Virtually all of them will have a desire to work with people in a helping profession.

My writing style in this book is personal and stylistically simple. I value short, clear sentences over a scholarly writing style. Writing style also bears on an issue that is sometimes a problem in clinical courses. The students almost universally want practical, applied knowledge more than they want scholarly writing. Most of the books in psychology and related fields are more formal in style than is *Clinical Practice with Adolescents*. In this book my first goal is to be useful. This practicality, however, is presented in the context of research that supports the useful content. Clinical courses are almost always taught by full-time faculty or by adjunct faculty drawn from practicing professionals. They are almost never taught by teaching assistants. Most instructors are more clinically oriented than research oriented, but they want a respectably serious style. My writing style balances a personal and practical tone with a solid research base.

In addition to the use of *Clinical Practice with Adolescents* in academia, any practitioner who deals with adolescents will find this book attractive as a basic reference and source of background. Clinics, hospitals, treatment centers, school psychology and counseling settings, and private practitioners will be able to use this book as a basic tool for clinical practice.

ABOUT THE AUTHOR

David G. Martin is professor of clinical psychology at the University of Manitoba, where he has been teaching for over 30 years. He is the author of five books in psychology and has edited one book. He has won three teaching awards as a university professor. Most of Dr. Martin's professional work is in the area of counseling and psychotherapy. He counsels clients himself and trains future clinical psychologists in counseling and therapy. In 1995 Dr. Martin received the Clifford Robson Distinguished Psychologist in Manitoba Award.

Most of Dr. Martin's clinical work is with adolescents. He does individual and group therapy and has supervised both group and individual therapy with adolescent clients. This interest in adolescence has been an important focus of Dr. Martin's career since the 1960s. His Ph.D. was earned at the University of Chicago, and his clinical internship was at the Institute for Juvenile Research in Chicago. While there, he completed his dissertation, titled "Consistency of self-descriptions under different role sets among neurotic and normal adolescents and adults."

WORKING WITH ADOLESCENTS

In this brief chapter I discuss the difficulties and rewards of working with troubled adolescents in order to help you decide whether you are among the minority of clinicians who both enjoy and do well with this age group. Also in this chapter I mention some of the most important psychological issues that affect clinical work with teenagers.

THE CHALLENGE OF CLINICAL WORK WITH ADOLESCENTS

"Only the most courageous, or perhaps the most foolish, therapists are willing to treat adolescents, for they are the most difficult group of children with whom to work. Still, successes can be very rewarding in spite of the difficulties one encounters in working with them" (Spiegel, 1996, p. 130). Spiegel knows what he is talking about, but I have not quoted him to discourage you. My experience is that most clinicians do not like working with adolescent clients, but a few clinicians just seem to connect well with this age group, and you might be one of them. Liddle (1995) notes that "many studies and reviews of the literature reached the same conclusion: engaging adolescents in outpatient therapy presents extraordinary clinical challenges and fails with alarming frequency" (p. 39). This alarming failure rate has mostly to do with getting teenagers to participate in treatment in the first place and then with keeping them in treatment. If you can accomplish this, there are many techniques and interventions that can be helpful, but they cannot be helpful unless you first connect with the adolescent. As you read this book, you should always be thinking about the personal questions, "Am I one of the minority who can connect with teenagers, and do I enjoy connecting with them?"

THE THREE R'S OF CLINICAL WORK WITH ADOLESCENTS: RELATIONSHIP, RELATIONSHIP, AND RELATIONSHIP

There is a recurring theme throughout this book. The practicing clinician needs to know a great deal about techniques, personal dynamics, the nature and causes of behavior disorders, and many other topics. However, all of the brilliantly understood knowledge in the world will not make a clinician effective with adolescent clients unless he or she is able to form good relationships with those clients. No matter what your approach to therapy is, it will not work unless your client is actively involved in the process (Bohart & Tallman, 1999). In fact, if your client is actively involved in the process, there are probably dozens of approaches, methods, and techniques that will be beneficial. The best predictor of successful treatment is the quality of the therapeutic relationship. A good relationship is almost certainly healing in and of itself, but it is also powerful because it contributes to keeping the client actively involved in the treatment process.

Techniques and methods are important, but they will not work without the three most important elements of treatment: relationship, relationship, and relationship. This is probably true of all kinds of psychological treatment, but it applies especially to working with adolescents (Sommers-Flanagan & Sommers-Flanagan, 1997; Morris & Nicholson, 1993; Reinecke, 1993), largely because, in general, adolescents have trouble trusting that adults will not judge them or try to take away their growing independence and autonomy.

Adolescents Are Not Just Slightly Smaller Adults

One difficulty that adults often have in understanding adolescents is that adults judge the adolescents as though they had the same psychological dynamics and needs as adults. Every adult was once an adolescent, but it still seems as though adults and adolescents are members of different cultures who barely share the same language. A common mistake adults make is to think of adolescent behavior in terms of what they themselves would and should do. Another potential mistake is to use the adult's (inevitably distorted) memories of how he or she was as an adolescent. Adolescent culture changes constantly (partly as a defense against the intrusion of adults), and few adolescents are impressed by such statements as "I remember perfectly well when I was your age . . ."

The Potential for Changing Lives

In many ways adolescence is the time of life when long-lasting change is most likely to occur. The young person is defining who he or she is and is just in the middle of the process of shaking off old influences and trying to become an autonomous adult. Treating younger children is often frustrating because they are so enmeshed in a destructive environment that seems to undo any good you can do. On the other hand, many disorders become more entrenched and difficult to treat as they become part of an adult adjustment. Working with adolescents is challenging and difficult, but there will be many times when you can briefly enter a young person's life and help him or her change the direction of that life in ways that will have an impact for many years.

Taking Care of the Clinician's Needs Too

Working with adolescent clients is both difficult and rewarding. Many of your rewards will be external, of course, such as being paid, but other rewards will be intrinsic to the process of helping adolescents change in positive ways. (I cannot repeat enough, if you do not find this process intrinsically rewarding, you really should not be in this line of work.)

The stresses of working with adolescent clients, however, are also many and strong, and it will be important that you always have in your life ways to help you deal with these stresses. You will be frustrated by young clients who seem to like you at some times and then inexplicably take offense with your fundamentally flawed character and inability to understand anybody, all in response to something you have done that seemed innocent and inconsequential at the time. Sometimes your clients will simply disappear from the radar screen, and adolescent clients frequently fail to show up for sessions.

Most clinical work with adolescents is probably done in interdisciplinary settings where no one person is entirely responsible for treatment. This shared responsibility takes some of the pressure off individual clinicians and provides the opportunity to build a network of support for yourself. You will be wise to establish a close, supportive relationship with one or a few colleagues. If you end up in private practice with adolescent clients, you should find a way to establish your own network of professional colleagues.

ADOLESCENT DEVELOPMENT

If you are interested in clinical work with adolescents, you should read extensively about adolescent personality development and adolescent culture; that literature is too vast to summarize here, of course. I have chosen to describe in this chapter a few aspects of adolescent development that bear strongly on your practice as a clinician.

The Myth of Adolescence as a Time of Turmoil and Pathology

Since the beginning of the 20th century (Hall, 1904; Freud, 1936/ 1946, 1969; Blos, 1962), mental health professionals have developed and promoted a view of adolescence, including normal adolescence, as a time of emotional instability, pathology, excessive egoism, and crisis. This viewpoint was based almost entirely on clinical impressions formed by therapists working with adolescent patients. Evidence from more systematic study of adolescents strongly contradicts this "all adolescents are disturbed anyway" viewpoint (Walsh & Paulson, 1994; Weiner, 1992), but this belief is still distressingly widely held among members of the public and among professionals.

The belief that adolescence is normally pathological has several unfortunate effects. First, it leads to a belief that we cannot really distinguish normal from abnormal behavior among adolescents. In fact, most adolescents are emotionally stable and mature in a continuous and gradual way without major disturbance (Petersen, 1988; Powers, Hauser, & Kilner, 1989). If clinicians have a tendency to dismiss abnormal behavior as just the way teenagers are, they will falsely ignore problems that really are problems and can be treated. A second and related false belief is that deviant behavior in adolescents is normative and therefore that they will just grow out of it.

The most insidious effect of the "adolescence is a time of disturbance" belief is its impact on the clinician's fundamental attitude toward adolescents. Successful clinicians are not naively optimistic, but they do have an underlying attitude that adolescents in general are interesting people who are trying to live as well as they can and are entirely capable of positive change under the right circumstances. If you believe, even unconsciously, that adolescents (and especially adolescent clients) are fundamentally flawed and need to be fixed, you will probably have difficulty forming the kind of personal connections that make clinical contact with adolescents work.

Being Aware of the Individual's Level of Development

The needs and personality dynamics of early adolescence are different from those of middle or late adolescence. For example, the earlier years are probably focused more on establishing independence and autonomy, whereas the later years are more likely to involve establishing intimacy with potential romantic partners. Any individual adolescent might be in the "early years" at age 13, and another could have the concerns of the "early years" at age 18. Because adolescence is a time of rapid change, the clinician must be alert and sensitive to the needs of the client as an individual with a specific set of needs.

Special Psychological Needs

This is not a textbook on adolescent psychology, but several developmental tasks are especially important in adolescence, and the clinician needs to understand these in order to work with this age group. These tasks are normal, important, and common, and an understanding of them will inform much of what you do with your clients. For example, if you understand the adolescent's intense need for autonomy, you will be much more sensitive to your behaviors that might seem quite benign and innocent to you but that might be perceived by the client as another adult trying to control him or her.

Need for Independence and Autonomy   Adolescents have a strong need to feel empowered. The special psychological need of adolescents that will have the greatest effect on you as a clinician is the adolescent's need to be in control of his or her life. You will be trying to have a significant and helpful impact on your clients, but you need to find ways to have this influence without being perceived by your adolescent clients as controlling, judgmental, and a threat to their autonomy. In general, adolescents expect adults to be controlling and judgmental and are poised to resist. It is important for therapists to trust their adolescent clients' capacity to solve problems and grow, and it is important to communicate this trust to your client in whatever way you can. The effective clinician implies in many ways, "I am not going to try to control you. You control you. I want to help you find good ways to do that."

Need to Belong   One of the most important ways that adolescents define their own identity is through their identification with a group. Adolescent culture is marked by the importance of identity groups of many different kinds that provide most adolescents with a place to belong. This place to belong primarily involves peer relationships, partly because of the adolescent's need to break away from a lifetime of connection with the family. For almost all adolescents it is overwhelmingly important to feel accepted *somewhere.* Even if it means risking rejection by the majority of people, acceptance within a group is often worth adopting styles and behaviors that might seem odd or destructive to adults. Knowing this goes a long way toward helping a therapist not judge these behaviors and understand that they serve a purpose. This does not imply a passive acceptance of what might even be dangerous behaviors, but it does encourage an acceptance of the adolescent. This knowledge also guides the therapist toward providing the kinds of belonging that can help clients find better places to belong, for example, in group programs or in new sets of friends.

Need to Be Different/Need to Be the Same   Two of the adolescent's strongest needs inherently conflict with each other. The need for independence and autonomy often means that it is important to be different and unique. On the other hand, the need to be accepted by others almost always requires some conformity and being similar to others. This creates a confusing and sometimes painful dilemma for adolescents. The clinician who understands, accepts, and responds to this principle is far more likely to be sensitive to and to understand some of the apparent capriciousness of adolescent behavior. It is often important for the adolescent client to discover, with the clinician's help and acceptance, that having conflicting needs is pretty normal and that there are ways to be both unique and accepted at the same time. Discovering a way to balance and accept this important conflict is a good opportunity to learn about balancing and accepting conflicting needs in general—a terribly important lesson.

Separation from Parents (and Other Adults)   It is often said that an adolescent's greatest need is not to need his or her parents anymore, but the parents' greatest need is still to be needed. This sets up an almost inevitable conflict between the two sets of needs. The adolescent's need to get rid of his or her parents emotionally is obviously partly an extension of the general need for independence and autonomy. Becoming independent from parents, however, is an especially difficult problem because so many years of a different kind of relationship have to be undone. The child has been both dependent on and subordinate to the parents in many ways, and replacing the old relationship with a new relationship is often a painful and wrenching process that is frequently marked by hostile feelings.

There are, of course, many possible sources of these hostile feelings. Many parents base their relationships with their young children on power rather than on the firm and loving approach that sets clear limits but also takes the child's needs and input into account (Maccoby & Martin, 1983). Autocratic parents clearly lose most of their power when their children become adolescents and start fighting back in the same power-based, adversarial way they have been treated. Although this rebellion against authority certainly leads to a lot of unpleasantness between adolescents and parents, even the most firm and loving parent is likely to be rejected in some painful ways as the child enters adolescence. The adolescent has to weaken some of the strongest bonds of childhood in order to become autonomous. There probably is no easy way to do this.

I have to be careful not to exaggerate the picture of normal adolescence as a time of rebellion against parents, just as it is important not to see adolescence in general as a time of emotional disturbance. It does seem true that one normal task of adolescents is to separate from parents, but this is not necessarily a time of guerrilla warfare. Walsh and Paulson (1994) cite many studies that indicate that "adolescence is marked by an increase in familial conflict and a decrease in emotional attachment to parents, but these changes tend to be temporary, minor disruptions in the parent-child relationship. Furthermore, the conflicts tend to be minor disputes over mundane issues" (p. 152). Most teenagers separate relatively peacefully from their parents (Offer & Sabshin, 1984).

However, clinical work with adolescents selectively brings you into contact with the minority of young people who are struggling most with their relationships with parents. The clinician needs to understand that, as an adult, he or she is parent-like enough to arouse the adolescent's suspicion that the clinician is also a threat to independence and autonomy. It is important for the clinician to be supportive and collaborative in ways that do not shout "control."

Identity Issues   Erikson (1956) argued that the primary psychological task during adolescence was to form an identity, a clear and consistent definition of who the individual *is*. There is some evidence (Martin, 1969) that developing a consistent self-description is especially difficult for adolescents with emotional problems. Adolescents who were clients of a mental health clinic described their own personalities significantly differently in different situations and roles. Adolescents who were not receiving treatment were consistent in their self-descriptions in different roles, as were two groups of adults—those with emotional problems and those without. Some inconsistency of self-descriptions seems normal and even adaptive in some ways. Adolescents with emotional problems are unusually inconsistent in how they describe themselves. This knowledge helps a therapist to be sensitive to the inconsistencies in an adolescent's life and self-perceptions—not with the goal of making the adolescent consistent but to acknowledge, accept, and work with whatever inconsistency means in the client's life.

Need for a Sense of Purpose   Adolescents are especially sensitive to issues of meaning and purpose in life. They are likely to ask themselves frequently, "What's the point in anything?" This need also is often expressed through a heightened concern about fairness and unfairness. There are two implications of this for clinical practice. You will need to be alert to hear, encourage, and accept attempts to explore this search for meaning, and you will need to be as dependable and consistent as you can. For the adolescent, dependability in an adult is practically an ethical issue.

Need for Intimacy   During the later stages of adolescence, the focus starts to shift from being accepted by a group toward forming an intimate bond as part of a couple. Like the need to belong, the need for intimacy seems to be based on a hunger for acceptance.

Handling Sexuality   Any list of important issues for adolescents must include sexuality. The rapid development of the adolescent's sexuality can and will have important effects that many clinicians will miss, partly because young people tend to avoid talking about sex with adults and partly because many clinicians are not entirely comfortable with the topic themselves. Some clients will be bothered by guilt and anxiety about sex, and others will have trouble controlling their sexual behavior in ways that will cause them problems. Some will be caught up in a discovery of their attraction to members of the same sex, and most of them will have some fears about sex itself or the way society reacts to their sexuality. This is a difficult topic, and the sensitive clinician will be listening for ways to respond to it without being perceived as intrusive or pushy about it.

CULTURAL COMPETENCE IN AN AGE OF DIVERSITY

North America is rapidly becoming more culturally diverse. Many estimates predict that within 20 or 30 years Whites will be a numerical minority in the United States. In addition to racial diversity, ethnic and cultural diversity are already so common in our society that you may be called on to offer services to adolescents and their families who have backgrounds that are different from your own. It might be fairly straightforward to transfer much of the practice of medicine from one ethnic group to another, but the treatment of emotional problems is inherently linked to social norms.

In much of this book I devote space to the importance of helping clients feel understood, known, and accepted. This is difficult enough to do with an adolescent from your own culture. To do it well with teenagers from other cultures requires a great deal of new learning about those cultures, self-awareness of your own cultural biases, and an understanding of how culture bound most approaches to mental health are. From this perspective I have to admit that the information in this book is culture bound. For example, much of the treatment I talk about involves talking about problems and encouraging independence. Many Western readers would respond, "Well, of course it involves talking about problems and encouraging independence." That just seems natural and obvious, and it is difficult to be sensitive to how unnatural this might seem to someone from another culture. Some native American cultures, for example, see talkativeness as intrusive and personal independence as a violation of commitment to the good of the group.

Virtually all the popular approaches to treatment of adolescent problems have been developed by and for people of Western European descent. We must adapt our methods to help those from a wide variety of backgrounds. In this book I try to strike a balance between discussing specific activities you can use in your practice and explaining the principles behind those activities. Your primary focus should be on understanding the underlying principles so that you can adapt your practice to many settings and diverse individuals. It is usually rigid and wasteful to develop a set of techniques. If you understand the principles behind what you are doing, you will have thousands of techniques; in fact, you will probably have a different set of techniques for every person you work with, all based on the same principles. For example, if an underlying principle is that it is healing for a person to feel known and accepted by another, this might lead you to work with one adolescent by using verbal empathy, with another by sitting silently for long periods of time, and by playing cards or shooting baskets with another.

The Clinician's Self-Awareness

You and I are products of our cultures in ways that pervade our whole beings, ways that are so far-reaching and subtle that we can never fully understand them. Most people deny that they are particularly biased culturally, but this is an illusion for virtually all of us. It is possible, however, to increase your understanding of your own cultural heritage in ways that will enhance your clinical work.

The first step in developing your cultural self-awareness should be to describe your own background as thoroughly as possible for yourself. That means answering general questions, such as "What is my cultural heritage?" It also means articulating what groups you most strongly identify with, the traditions you practice and that seem natural to you, and the beliefs and attitudes you hold. A useful exercise is to name your dominant culture and then make a list of beliefs, assumptions, and values typical of that culture. Examine how committed you are to these values, beliefs, and assumptions.

The second step is an honest examination of your views of other ethnic groups. What is the source of these views? An honest answer will probably include the opinions of others from your own culture and family as a major source, and you need to ask what you have done to validate your views. Do you treat people from other ethnic groups differently because of their origin? An honest answer almost always includes some recognition of cultural bias in one's behavior. It sometimes helps to observe yourself interacting with people from other cultures, trying to be aware and sensitive to your own behavior that you might normally ignore. Things to watch for include whether you tell or enter into ethnic jokes or stereotypical comments, make statements of generalization about members of other cultures, or use derogatory terms to describe people who are culturally different.

Understanding Cultures

In addition to self-awareness, you should increase your knowledge of cultures of adolescents you are likely to treat. You can do this through formal study and reading, of course, but it is probably more useful to learn from direct experience with people from the other cultural groups. This can include your clients, but you can and should also seek out people and resources indigenous to the culture you are interested in.

Your goal is to acquire culture-specific knowledge, of course, but you must be careful not to generalize too freely from your necessarily limited new knowledge. It would obviously be silly to think that because you had talked extensively with a dozen people from Egypt, you have a good grasp of Egyptian culture.

The most useful approach as a practicing clinician is probably best described as humble receptiveness. It is almost certainly impossible to understand a culture completely without growing up in it. Try to become as culturally aware as possible, but communicate to your clients that, although you are really trying to understand, you will need their help with the parts of their culture that are subtle and important. If you try to act like an expert, you will almost certainly fail to be helpful.

Special Issues Raised by Culture

Vraniak and Pickett (1993) outline five specific issues that commonly affect treatment work with clients from minority groups. It is often said that adolescents in general come from a different culture than adults, so all five of these issues are common to work with most adolescents, but they are especially contentious with minority clients.

1. Children and adolescents from minority groups often have difficult and contentious relationships with authority figures. Thus the therapy relationship may be more difficult to form because trust will take longer to develop. A cultural norm in minority groups often is (for good reasons, historically) to hide from and mislead authority figures from the dominant group.
2. Minority clients often do things to test their clinicians' practical knowledge of their culture. Actually, adolescents in general do

this to adults, using terminology and referring to topics from their own culture to see whether the therapist or counselor is cool enough (knowledgeable enough) to be trusted and included. It is important to know as much as possible to pass these tests, but it is also important not to try to fake understanding. If you admit ignorance too much, you will lose credibility, but if you fake understanding, you absolutely will be caught and will lose both trust and credibility.

3. Clients will be especially interested in exploring knowledge about the clinician as a person and as an authority figure. Self-disclosure around issues of trust and authority is often needed. The fundamental principle that guides all self-disclosure in therapy is that it must be designed to benefit the client and not simply reflect the clinician's wish to talk.

4. It is more difficult for minority clients to perceive and believe that the clinician cares about them.

5. The treatment process is more likely to be unfamiliar to minority clients. The clinician probably will need to structure and explain the process more than with other clients. In addition, the treatment process needs to be adapted in ways that seem plausible and potentially helpful within the client's worldview.

The most important principle is to communicate a sensitivity to, understanding of, and willingness to work within the client's cultural perspective.

WORKING WITH ADOLESCENTS IS DIFFERENT

The best way to summarize this chapter is to say that working with adolescents is different from working with either children or adults. It takes a special kind of clinician, and it takes an understanding of and respect for adolescent culture.

Recommended Reading

McClure, F. H., & Teyber, E. (Eds.). (1996). *Child and adolescent therapy: A multicultural-relational approach.* Fort Worth: Harcourt Brace.

Prout, H. T., & Brown, D. T. (1999). *Counseling and psychotherapy with children and adolescents.* New York: Wiley.

Semrud-Clikeman, M. (1995). *Child and adolescent therapy.* Needham Heights, MA: Allyn and Bacon.

BUILDING AN ALLIANCE

More than in any other chapter, in this one I am concerned with what you will actually do with your adolescent client. In other chapters I give you background information and strategies for dealing with special situations. All the knowledge in the world, however, will not help you be an effective clinician with adolescents unless you know how to make a personal connection with your clients.

THE IMPORTANCE OF RELATIONSHIP

The central theme of this book is that many techniques of therapy are important and effective, but the most important element of successful therapy is the quality of the therapeutic relationship. Therapy is effective, but no one school of therapy is better than another; the best predictor of successful therapy is the therapeutic relationship. The evidence for this position is extensive when discussing therapy with clients of all ages (Najavits & Strupp, 1994; Whiston & Sexton, 1993), but it is especially important in doing therapy with adolescents (Sommers-Flanagan & Sommers-Flanagan, 1997; Morris & Nicholson, 1993; Reinecke, 1993).

Treating adolescents requires both a good relationship and an extremely creative and flexible use of techniques. One reason that doing therapy with adults is easier than doing therapy with adolescents is that adult clients have a general expectation that they will be seeing you in an office and that therapy will be based primarily on talking together for a limited period of time. Adolescent clients are much more wary, often cannot stand to sit still for an hour, and frequently find the process of just talking a little strange. All of this means that you will need a much broader set of relationship builders and techniques with adolescent clients. It is almost misleading to refer to what the therapist does with these clients as techniques, because there are so many hundreds of different things the therapist can do. The main point is that, no matter how clever and powerful your techniques are, you will have little or no impact on an adolescent client unless you first have a good relationship. A psychologist I knows says that, with adolescents, he thinks of the therapist's techniques as the important payload that will have no effect unless the therapist has a good delivery vehicle, which is a good relationship. Meeks (1997) says, "The first and most important part of developing a psychotherapeutic relationship with an adolescent patient is the evolution of a therapeutic alliance" (p. 381).

The Therapeutic Alliance

Because the therapy relationship is the most important part of therapy, many researchers are studying it, usually under the general term *therapeutic alliance.* Many different definitions and measures of therapeutic alliance are currently in use (Horvath & Luborsky, 1993), but two basic components of the alliance are included in all of them.

First, the *personal bond* between client and therapist includes the kind of characteristics that most people think of when they think of good relationships—personal warmth, empathy, and acceptance. This part of the alliance is fundamental throughout therapy, and it is probably most critical early in therapy when the client is establishing trust in the therapist. With adult clients, the "strength of therapeutic alliance is established within the first three sessions of psychotherapy with little significant change over the course of therapy" (Eaton, Abeles, & Gutfreund, 1988, p. 536). This is probably even more true with adolescent clients (Katz, 1990). It is unnerving but true that a lot is riding on your first contact with an adolescent client. Probably the two most important things that will establish an initial contact with your client is that she perceive you as being on her side and that she feels you clearly understand what she is trying to say. Most adolescents say, "Nobody listens to me," and they are generally right. They also usually have a strong expectation that an adult will approach them with corrective advice and at least some judgment. If you meet these expectations in your first contact with the adolescent, developing a personal bond will be difficult. Throughout this chapter I discuss many ways to establish this personal bond.

Second, in a good alliance both the client and the therapist have a *collaborative commitment* to the mutual work and goals of therapy. This part of the alliance is more task oriented. In general, the client and the therapist are in agreement about where they are going, and both of them see their work together as a collaboration rather than as something under the control of the therapist. The element of commitment is necessary for the client to be the active source of growth in therapy, and the therapist's commitment to the process is one of the most powerful ways that the therapist demonstrates that the client is valued and accepted. This aspect of the alliance is much easier to recognize and establish with adult clients than with adolescents. The process of therapy is less well defined with adolescents, and they are often skeptical of the procedures and structures that are usually involved in psychotherapy. Thus much of the attention in this book is on ways to get adolescent clients involved in and committed to the process.

Your Relationship as a Curative Environment

The therapeutic relationship may be the most powerful intervention available to us. Clinicians can interact with adolescent clients in dozens of ways, but the fundamental essence that underlies all these different ways of being in therapy is that the client feels *deeply known* and *accepted*. As clinicians, we are often impressed with our own techniques and interventions that, in fact, often are powerful and effective, but the success of our interventions depends on the alliance. Moreover, many times the things that make up a good relationship are in and of themselves healing. For example, the free and easy talking that results from being understood almost inevitably leads to effective problem solving. In addition, an adolescent who experiences acceptance from a person who deeply knows him or her comes to feel more self-acceptance without any other particular intervention. It really may be true that the connection heals.

If the essence of treatment is being deeply known and accepted, then the fundamental qualities that the clinician brings to the adolescent are *understanding* and *respect*. I have many things to say about how understanding and respect are communicated.

It's a Trust Thing   I once asked one of my adolescent clients about who was helpful and who was not helpful at the treatment center where he was receiving various kinds of help. The treatment center provided an interdisciplinary program, so the young man had had contact with a wide variety of clinicians. He thought carefully before he answered my question about what the difference was between helpful and unhelpful clinicians. He finally said, "It's a trust thing." He meant several things by this. He said, "You have to get to know the person. And they have to get to know you. Some of them expect you just to sit down in a room and open up. It just doesn't happen that way. When they are like who they really are, it seems more like they're a real person, not just getting paid to do a job. Then you're really who you are, telling them your real problem."

He made another point about workers he trusted. "That way they don't seem so critical. . . . It's more like they're giving advice." Helpful clinicians were consistently accepting of him as a person, even when they delivered consequences for unacceptable behavior. They listened and considered his point of view as having a reality that made sense to him, both when having positive interactions and when having disagreements. He was bothered by clinicians who seemed friendly and understanding at some times but, when they were frustrated, said things that felt like personal attacks that went beyond delivering consequences or just disagreeing with the young man. I think the key issue here was unpredictable criticism and judgment.

Providing Consistency   One important way that respect is communicated is through being dependable. No one is ever entirely consistent, but one of the most important things you can offer an adolescent client is to do what you say you are going to do and not switch back and forth in the fundamental ways that you relate to your client. Adolescents with emotional problems usually feel conflicted about their relationships with adults, largely because many adults fluctuate unpredictably between loving behaviors and punitive behaviors. This is often more damaging than adult behavior that is exclusively punitive. It is more confusing and harder to escape from a relationship that is unpredictably positive and negative.

Forthrightness   Adolescent clients are almost always wary of adults and are extremely sensitive to phoniness. A clinician needs to be as free as possible from expert role playing and as genuine as possible about acting naturally. Being forthright does not mean saying everything that's on your mind, but it does mean acting in ways that are consistent with who you really are.

Presence   One of the most powerful things that clinicians bring to the curative environment of the relationship is *presence.* Presence is difficult to define, but with an adolescent client it is probably best understood as a focused concentration on the client. If you are just there doing your job, you will have much less impact than if you really want to know your client's story. The client of a clinician with presence would say, for example, "He is really interested in what I have to say" or "She really pays attention to me."

Therapy is probably the only place where two people are focused on one person's experience, and the client usually feels the therapist's presence as an undistracted interest in what the client is dealing with. There is an intensity to presence, but it is a quietly strong intensity rather than a frenetic intensity.

Most Adolescents Expect Judgment from Adults

Not only do adolescents feel that adults do not listen to them, but they also expect adults to respond primarily with corrective advice, facile reassurance that essentially communicates the message, "Stop feeling the way you do because it doesn't make any sense," various intensities of scolding, or direct criticism and judgment. They are used to adults prefacing their responses with, "That may be, but . . . ," "Yes, but . . . ," and other lead-in comments that seem to imply some acknowledgment of what the adolescent has said. Adolescents, however, are seldom fooled by our attempts to disguise our judgments.

This unpleasant reality of the adolescent's world creates a powerful opportunity for the clinician who wants to connect with the adolescent. The adolescent is often pleasantly startled to meet an adult who does not judge him or her. This pleasant surprise contributes to trust, to a willingness to talk, and to the first steps in giving up the wariness with which most adolescents approach adults.

This does not mean that the clinician is permissive or approves of everything that the adolescent does. It does mean that the clinician proves to the adolescent that he or she has heard what the adolescent means and can understand how that meaning is important to the adolescent. Sommers-Flanagan and Sommers-Flanagan (1995) have a nice way of saying how to do this: "The solution is deceptively simple: side with the adolescent" (p. 133). This does not mean taking sides with the adolescent against others. It means wanting to know the adolescent's side and being committed to finding what's good for the adolescent. The clinician's responses give the client the following kinds of experiences: "She may not agree with me, but she really knows how things are for me" or "He really seems to know what I'm trying to say" or "He isn't trying to lay his own agenda on me, but he really cares that I figure things out and make my life better." This siding with the adolescent depends heavily on the clinician being deeply empathic and suspending judgment.

I hope that the previous paragraph relieved some of your possible, and understandable, worries that responding to an adolescent in a nonjudgmental way might reinforce unacceptable behaviors, partly by making the adolescent think that you agree with those behaviors. The subtle and powerful skill that you need is to make the other person feel understood and accepted as a person without either condoning or condemning his or her behaviors. This helps the person understand and accept him- or herself and come up with his or her own answers. It proves to the teenager the reality and power of his or her personal autonomy, and it proves that the therapist values, believes in, and encourages that autonomy.

Meeks (1997, p. 382) also has some useful advice for the clinician.

> Often the youngsters expect the therapist to be moralistic or to try to control their behavior; sometimes they expect the therapist to behave like a teacher asking for performance and judging the quality of that output. Frequently they expect the therapist to try to act superior to them to demonstrate the greater power that is associated with adulthood. When the adolescent makes these accusations directly, it is probably most useful just to agree that if therapy worked in that way, it would indeed be unacceptable. If it is possible to question the perception without appearing overly defensive or argumentative, that is usually wise also. For example, when the adolescent is reasonably calm, the therapist can ask: "Can you help me with that? Explain what I said or did that led you to believe that I'm trying to tell you what to do."

GETTING STARTED

Early Sessions Are Crucial

One of the most striking findings in the research on the therapeutic alliance is that the client's perception of a good relationship as early as the third interview is a strong predictor of eventual outcome. Even more striking is the earlier conclusion that the "strength of therapeutic alliance is established within the first three sessions of psychotherapy with little significant change over the course of therapy" (Eaton, Abeles, & Gutfreund, 1988, p. 536). Most of this evidence was gathered with adult clients, but it is extremely easy to lose adolescent clients in the first two or three sessions because of their difficulty in trusting adults and their vigilant sensitivity to betrayals of that trust through misunderstanding and judgment.

Sometimes, even the first few minutes are critical. Katz (1990) writes that "a number of opportunities to engage or repel the adolescent patient may occur during the first few minutes of the first interview. Those opening moments, the dynamics involved, and the tactics available require special attention" (p. 69). Katz has a number of suggestions for increasing the chances that those first few minutes will help you form a connection. One suggestion is that you quickly put into words thoughts that are uppermost on the client's mind. For example, you might anticipate the client's apprehension and possible reluctance about seeing a clinician. If you sense distrust from your client, it is important to articulate and accept that distrust and to let the client know "that I know that I am a stranger to him, that he does not know what I am like, and that he has no reason to trust me, and, indeed, that there would be something wrong if he did immediately trust a stranger" (Katz, 1990, p. 74). Another possible strategy that Katz suggests is to join with the client to analyze the situation together. This focuses attention outside the client and on the situation and lets the clinician and the client collaborate on something less threatening than examining the client's experiences. Meeks (1997) says that "the key element in developing a therapeutic alliance is the capacity to respond empathically to the adolescent's resistances to the very process of therapy and to recognize and respond to elements of negative transference as they begin to appear in the interaction with the therapist" (p. 382). Your adolescent client will almost inevitably be suspicious of you as an adult. An early understanding and affirmation of the wisdom of this wariness will go far to start building your therapeutic alliance.

Understanding the Adolescent's Starting Point

An important attitude that the clinician brings to the first few minutes of contact with an adolescent client is an open receptiveness and a lack of strongly held preconceptions. Katz (1998) gives an important reminder when he says, "In working with difficult patients, it is helpful to remember that the patient who comes into a psychiatrist's office only occasionally resembles the description given by parents, referring doctors, social workers, and so forth" (p. 90). This observation is consistent with the experiences of most clinicians I know. It is usually helpful to be familiar with a potential client's clinical file ahead of time, but there is also a danger involved because every report and assessment in the file is filtered through the perspective and needs and inevitable distortions of the person who wrote the report. Many clinicians approach their adolescent client with an already formed picture of the client and his or her problems. This can be helpful if it tunes the clinician in to potential problems in a way that helps in knowing the client better and more quickly. The obvious problem is that strongly held preconceptions can lead the clinician to a distorted understanding of what the client is trying to say and can contribute to the creation of self-fulfilling prophecies.

Katz also says that "the establishment of the therapeutic alliance does not always start with the first encounter between patient and therapist. There is often a preset relationship that the patient has developed with a fantasied therapist" (p. 89). This is another issue that demands that the clinician remain open and sharply attuned to what the client is saying in their first encounter rather than to what the clinician expects the client to be thinking and anticipating. Your client may even have expectations and fantasies about you as an individual, perhaps based on your reputation among other adolescents, and he or she will certainly have expectations and fantasies about you as a clinician in general. This may be based on cultural stereotypes about clinicians, or it may be based on previous experiences the adolescent has had with other clinicians. Sometimes this can work in your favor, especially if the previous experience was good, but there almost always is a price to pay. If the previous experience was a negative one, you will have ground to make up, and if the previous experience was very positive, you will have a lot to live up to. All of this is part of tuning in to the client's starting point and being open to wherever that is.

A clinician I know often says, "If you want to get from Point A to Point B with your client, you better first go to Point A." This is true throughout the treatment relationship, but it is probably the most true in your first contact with your client.

What's in This for the Adolescent?

One of the most important things that happens at the beginning of therapy is for the client to feel motivated to commit to the process. Nearly all adolescent clients approach treatment with some apprehension and reluctance. Many of them, of course, have been forced into therapy, at least in their perception. Even those who willingly enter a relationship with a clinician are usually confused about the nature of the process and worried about their loss of autonomy. In some way the client needs to understand the answer to the questions "Why should I do this, and what's in this for me?"

At some point early in treatment, I like to say something that conveys the message, "Our purpose together is to try to find some way to make your life better in a way that makes sense to you." Another way to get the message across might be, "I'd like to understand the things in your life that you wish were different and to see if we can figure out some way to make them different." My purpose is to help the client see that he or she has something to gain from the process, to create an atmosphere of mutual problem solving, and to relieve some of the client's fear that something is about to be imposed on him or her.

EMPATHY: ESTABLISHING A BOND WITH RESPECT AND UNDERSTANDING

The first element of the therapeutic alliance is the formation of a personal bond. Although there is much about the ability to form a bond that cannot be explained in a book, some skills can be described.

Clinicians must learn many things to be effective. The absolute foundation ability, however, is being able to make another person feel deeply understood. There are many names for this ability, but the most common one is *empathy*. The problem is that many people misunderstand empathy to be some kind of warm and supportive reflection of what the client has just said. Paraphrasing what the other person has said often does make the other person feel understood. Sometimes, however, it does not. There is no one skill or technique that constitutes empathy. Empathy can be anything you do that gives the other person the experience that "you really under-stood what I meant."

This kind of understanding consists of two major elements. First, you must understand what the other person *meant,* and this especially involves hearing what was implied by the other person. Second, you must communicate this understanding to the other person in some way that helps them experience, "Yes, exactly, that is what I was trying to say."

Like most things in therapy, hearing what the other person meant—the intended message—is more difficult with adolescents than with adult clients. When it comes to communicating your un-derstanding of the intended message, the gap between adult and adolescent clients is even larger. Making an adolescent feel under-stood often requires far more than a well-worded verbal response.

Hearing the Intended Message

The first step in deep listening is to tune in sensitively to what the person *means.* In spoken English the words used carry much less than half the meaning intended in the communication. The bulk of the meaning is carried through tone, expression, context, and, most important, what is implied by the words used. There is a fine line be-tween hearing what another person means and going beyond what the person intended for you to hear into your own interpretations of what you judge the other person's psychological dynamics to be. Hearing the intended message certainly requires you to draw infer-ences, to sense emotions that may or may not be explicitly expressed, and to find meaning beyond the actual words used. All these sen-sitive skills, however, are used in the service of *what the other per-son wants you to hear.*

This sensitive attunement to another person is difficult enough with adult clients, as I have discussed elsewhere (Martin, 2000). Adolescent clients, however, are usually even less explicit and clear in their expression of meaning than adults. They often speak in a code that is always changing and is intended to isolate and exclude adults while helping the adolescent feel more a part of his or her own peer culture. The therapist usually cannot use this adolescent code language without looking like an adolescent wannabe, but the therapist usually needs to understand the code to be a good lis-tener. In some ways, I think that adolescent clients often use this language to test their therapists, to see if the therapist really does understand and is cool enough to be trusted to listen.

It is not only the special language of adolescents that requires the therapist to listen sensitively. All of us have some difficulty explicitly expressing our real thoughts, especially when they involve emotion. Adolescents tend to be less psychologically minded than adults and especially less psychologically minded than adults who are clinicians. An adolescent client might say, "English sucks." This could mean a dozen different things. Your job is to understand whether this utterance means that English is difficult, the teacher is mean, the teacher is strict, the client is angry, the client feels hopeless, the client is bored because English is too easy, or any of the other different meanings that the phrase could have. Your goal is to understand in a way that, when you communicate your understanding, your client will feel, "Exactly right. That's what I meant." If you can help your client feel this way, you will have taken one more step in making it easy for your client to talk to you.

Communicating Your Understanding

For now, let's assume that you have correctly heard and understood what your client meant for you to hear and understand, including the implied feelings. How do you prove to your client that you have heard and understood all of this? Many books on counseling and therapy suggest a response that usually goes something like, "It sounds like you feel . . ." and the counselor puts into his or her own words what the other person has implied. This kind of response is often helpful and, when done well, can make the other person feel deeply understood. There is a danger, however, that people will come to think of this kind of response as the only kind that qualifies as a good empathic response. What qualifies as a good empathic response is anything you say or do that makes your client feel deeply understood and known. This is the absolute essence of empathy, and there are dozens of ways to make a person feel deeply understood.

This was cleverly demonstrated in a study by Bachelor (1988). Bachelor asked clients to describe "a situation in which your therapist was empathic toward you (i.e., when you felt that he or she demonstrated the ability to put himself or herself in your place). Write in detail what happened and what you felt" (p. 229). Bachelor found that many kinds of therapist responses were reported as "received empathy" that made the client feel understood. The therapist response that most often was perceived as empathic was *therapist (facilitative) cognitive empathy.* This is the kind of response I

discussed in the previous paragraph; the therapist expresses—verbally and nonverbally—his or her understanding of what the client
was trying to say. Other kinds of therapist responses, however, were
also sometimes perceived as deeply empathic. *Therapist affective
empathy* included experiences in which the therapist personally experienced emotions that the client was experiencing. Sometimes
therapist sharing empathy was perceived as deeply empathic when
the therapist spontaneously shared personal opinions or personal
experiences that related to what the client was saying. Although
more rare, *therapist nurturant empathy* sometimes occurred when
the therapist expressed direct support, attention, and acceptance.
Sometimes even advice or interpretations are perceived as deeply
empathic by a client. It would be wrong to say that it doesn't matter what the therapist does, but it is important that we understand
that there are many ways to make a person feel understood. The absolute essence of powerful, effective listening is that the client feels
deeply known.

If there are dozens of ways to make an adult client feel understood, there must be three times that many ways of expressing understanding to an adolescent. My experience is that most of the time
with most adolescents it is helpful to respond with leading phrases,
such as "It sounds like you feel . . . ," "I get the sense that the part
of this that bothers you most has something to do with your dad,"
"If you could have things just the way you want them, my guess is
that nobody would be required to go to school," or any of the hundreds of ways that you can put into words what the other person
has implied. Many times, however, less direct expressions of understanding are more effective with adolescents. I discuss several
of these ways to express understanding, but I want to be careful
that you do not see this as a list of techniques. Do not lose sight of
the essence of deep listening; these suggestions are useful only if
they serve the purpose of making the other person feel deeply
understood.

Let's contrast the therapist response that helps the client feel
"Exactly!" with some of the other ways that adults respond to adolescents—ways that make it less likely that the client will find the
adult easy to talk to. In an interpretation the adult might say, "The
reason you think English sucks is that you are afraid of failing in
English." This may or may not be correct, but it is the adult's "wiser,
more sophisticated" understanding that the adult is using to explain where the client "is wrong." If this is not what the client meant
for the clinician to hear, there are many things the adolescent might

say in response, but I promise you that he or she will be a little less likely to tell the therapist things that matter. Many adults would have responded to "English sucks" with corrective advice: "I think you would find English much more fun if you put just a little more work into it." Some would use facile reassurance: "Lots of kids don't like English very much. I'm sure you'll be okay in it." Some would use explicitly critical judgment: "The problem is not with English; the problem is that you're lazy."

Interpretation, constructive advice, reassurance, and even critical judgment often have a valid place in human relationships, including relationships with adolescents. In fact, I discuss ways that interpretations can be useful in therapy with adolescents. These kinds of communication are, however, almost always a barrier to forming a collaborative connection with another person, especially with adolescents.

Self-Disclosure   Letting your client know something about you is far more important with adolescent clients than it is with adult clients. It is more likely for an adult client to expect not to know much about his or her therapist and for the focus to be almost exclusively on the client. Because trust and relationship are so much more fragile and difficult with adolescent clients, the therapist's willingness to be known is much more important. Done skillfully, self-disclosure both helps build the therapeutic alliance and is a vehicle for helping your client feel more understood and accepted. There are, however, real risks in self-disclosure, so it is important that we understand the principles that make self-disclosure helpful.

Sharing your interests and experiences can make your clients feel valued enough that you trust them with this information. You are letting yourself be known by the client, and that implies some willingness to be vulnerable on your part. In addition, a story about yourself can imply an understanding of your client's experience in much the same way that talking about another teenager can get a point across without targeting the adolescent so directly that it threatens him or her. It is important, however, that your story be presented simply as your experience and that it not imply or directly state "I know just how you feel, because when I was your age . . ." The phrase "I know just how you feel" almost always backfires because the other person correctly feels that you are trivializing the uniqueness of his or her experience. It is better to tell your story with the implication of "I'm not exactly sure what that was like for you, but here's an experience of mine that may have some similarity."

re with adolescent clients has two major dangers.
elf-disclosure can violate appropriate interpersonal
ays that can make your client uncomfortable and
.... can inappropriately compromise your own privacy and
the privacy of other people in your life. The second potential problem is that the therapist may unwittingly be using self-disclosure
to meet his or her own personal needs. These needs can include a
wish to impress the client, an attempt to deal with some personal
issue of the therapist's, or even the enjoyment of having a chance
to talk about oneself. The essential principle is that the therapist
should be able to explain how any particular self-disclosure serves
the needs of the client.

Using Empathic Questions   Questions can serve many purposes,
and they seem to be more useful with adolescent clients than with
adult clients. In chapter 3 I discuss the use of questions in a way
that helps the adolescent client structure and focus the treatment
process. For now, though, I want to look at one kind of question that
is especially powerful in helping another person to feel understood:
empathic questions.

Most questions are designed to get information from the other
person, but empathic questions convey an understanding of what
the person was trying to say while giving the other person the opportunity to agree or disagree more easily than if the therapist's response had been made as a statement. Sometimes an expression of
empathic understanding that is worded as a question feels gentler
to the client. If my client were to say, "I kept trying to make myself
go home last night, but I thought my dad might be there," I could
respond in many different ways. I might gently ask, "Were you
scared?" This question is really only a question in grammatical form
and carries the same meaning as if I had said, "It sounds to me like
you were scared." Under some circumstances, however, the empathic question could be more respectful of the level of the client's
fear and could be perceived by the client as more understanding
but tentative.

An empathic question is often the best way to word a response
when you think you might be somewhat ahead of where the client
is and think you understand but aren't sure. The understanding-
but-tentative quality of your empathic question makes it clear to
your client that you are not trying to impose something on him or
her but are exploring with the client and that you really want to understand what he or she is experiencing. Empathic questions can

also give the client emotional permission to talk about difficult material. If you can tell that your client is trying to tell you something that is embarrassing or frightening or painful and that he or she just cannot get the words out, but both of you have a pretty good idea of where the story is going, it can be an enormous relief for you just to ask about the story in a calm, accepting way.

Using the Third Person   Sometimes adolescent clients have difficulty with direct responses to what they have said about themselves, but it is possible to express understanding of their experience by couching it in terms that refer to people in general or to other individuals. A client might say, "It's really stupid how everybody is supposed to have a boyfriend or a girlfriend." There are many ways a therapist could respond to this, such as, "I guess it really bothers you to be under that kind of pressure." Many adolescents, however, would feel that this was hitting too close to home, and if I thought my client might feel threatened by it, I could more gently say, "I guess a lot of kids hate the pressure that you always have to be going out with somebody."

Metaphors   Metaphors are often powerful ways to show understanding and can convey a great deal in a few words and even express complex experiential meaning quickly and in such a way that other words cannot (Cirillo & Crider, 1995). Angus and Rennie (1989) gathered evidence that suggested that "a metaphor is typically embedded within experiential networks of memories, incidents, images, and feelings constituting an 'associated meaning context'" (p. 377).

Adolescents often find metaphors easier to accept from the clinician than more direct statements. "That was a real kick in the gut" or "It's like he's the biggest gorilla in the jungle and you're small and trying to hide" or "It seems like other people think you're the biggest gorilla in the jungle, but they can't really see you for what you are" are three examples of the millions of metaphors that can help your client feel more understood. A few clinicians I have known seemed to go metaphor crazy, and this often strikes adolescents as slightly strange. Be careful that your metaphors make sense to your client.

Music Lyrics and Film Plots   An adolescent client and I were once driving in my car, listening to rap music (I will say more about car therapy in chapter 3), when he suddenly said, "That's how I used to be." I hadn't been listening to the lyrics of the music and was a bit confused for several seconds. It soon became clear, however, that the lyrics were speaking of an intense, fundamental, and uncontrolled rage. We rewound the tape and listened to the lyrics several times. Simply by saying, "That's how I used to be," my client had found a way to express feelings he had never been able to express before and to say a great deal about the progress he felt he had made in dealing with his anger. From then on, the lyrics to that rap song became an important part of how we talked about his anger. Weeks later, I could say, "Was this like that song?" He would respond, "A little, but I could have stopped." We had developed a mutual shorthand that no one else could have understood if they had been listening to it; having the music lyrics gave us a way to understand a complex experience and to share that understanding with only a few words.

A clinician who works with adolescents should have some familiarity with current music and with film plots that are likely to be important to their adolescent clients. Being able to say, "That's like what Darth Vader might do" can serve as a powerful expression of understanding that is expressed somewhat indirectly.

Nobody Ever Listens to Me

Most of the adolescents I have known have expressed some version of the thought that nobody ever listens to them. We adults often dismiss this as little more than adolescent complaining, but there probably is a lot of truth in it. [In fact, there is evidence that adults do not listen to each other very well either (Carkhuff & Berenson, 1977), but dealing with that would require another book.] I noted earlier that adults often respond to adolescents with various forms of judgment; it seems fair to say that we can broaden this to include a lack of real listening. Almost everyone is hungry to be listened to, and this certainly includes most adolescents. I hope for you that you know exactly what I am talking about, because you have experienced the feeling of having someone understand what you really mean, even when you were having trouble expressing yourself. The relief or pleasant surprise or even little rush of being understood like this has the compelling quality of making us want to say more. This hunger creates another opportunity for you to connect with a client.

Rogers (1980) gives a helpful description of how clients react to different levels of understanding. "If the therapist has communicated a superficial understanding of the client's expression, the client's inner response and perhaps verbal response will be, 'Of course. That's what I just said'" (p. 2155). Adolescent clients are likely to be less polite than this and may say, "Well, duh!" in response to superficial understanding in which the clinician pretty much repeats back what the client has just said instead of understanding what the client meant. One mother who was trying to understand her teenage daughter but who hadn't mastered this told me her daughter finally said, "Mother, what's wrong with you? You've gone crazy! All you ever do is repeat back what I just said." Rogers continues, "When the therapist has communicated an effectively empathic response, the client's reaction is likely to be, 'That's exactly right! I didn't suppose anyone could understand what I really meant. Now I wish to tell you some more'" (p. 2155). Being deeply understood by someone creates an almost irresistible draw to say more.

Being Known by Someone

A psychiatrist I know was being introduced to someone by a 16-year-old girl he was seeing in therapy. She described him to the other person as "the guy who knows me." I cannot think of a more meaningful compliment from a client than to be thought of this way, and her comment highlights for us something that is close to the essence of therapy: For a client to be deeply known, including her faults and weaknesses, by someone who still finds her interesting, valuable, and acceptable creates an enormous sense of safety and an environment in which the client is free to explore and change.

Good therapists often hear clients say, "You know me better than anyone else." I would hope for the person that a spouse or friend or someone else from real life would be the person who knows the client best, but that is often not the case, and being deeply known by a therapist can be a source of healing. It is important to understand that there are many ways to make a person feel deeply known. Think back to the discussion of how many different ways there are to express understanding. Your goal is not to produce lots of good empathy responses; your goal is to help your client feel known.

Affirming Your Client

One of the most powerful effects of empathy is the experience that if someone else can understand what you are going through, what you are trying to say, how you view yourself, and how you view the world, it affirms your validity as a person. Who you *are* must make sense in some way, or the other person couldn't understand. The other person may even disagree with you, but you can still feel affirmed.

This is especially important when your adolescent client is trying to describe some personal characteristic that is often misunderstood by others. The clinician might say, "You get called lazy a lot, but I think you see yourself as a person who is trying really hard."

Respect and Understanding Are Not Agreement

Some clinicians worry that affirming their clients through understanding might somehow reinforce them for continuing to hold distorted ideas or to think that the clinician is approving of or agreeing with what they have said. But that is not the function of empathy. The good listener is communicating, "I understand your experience." The comment about trying hard made by the clinician in the previous paragraph neither approved nor disapproved and neither agreed nor disagreed with what the client had said.

Respect and Understanding Are Not Permissiveness

Another misunderstanding that some therapists have about basing treatment on respect and understanding is that the therapist is somehow being sweet, passive, and permissive. Making another person feel understood is none of these. The process of deep listening is active, evocative, and intense, and it is done within the context of consistent, reliable limits. Throughout this book I will have much to say about the context and limits of therapy, but it is important to be clear now that giving an adolescent the experience of being deeply known is not permissive.

Respect and Understanding Are Not Sympathy

It is common to confuse empathy with many other attributes, probably most often with sympathy. Sympathy implies pity. It says, "Oh, you poor thing; I feel sorry for you." Empathy implies trust. It says to the client that he or she is strong enough to solve problems, that the clinician will not condescend pityingly, and that the work they are doing together is hard work but within reach.

ESTABLISHING A COLLABORATIVE COMMITMENT

I have been discussing the first element of a good therapeutic alliance, forming a personal bond. The second element of a good therapeutic alliance focuses more on the work to be done together. Much of this work, of course, grows directly out of the formation of the personal bond, but now I want to focus more on treatment as a process of collaborative problem solving.

Horvath and Luborsky (1993) suggest that a collaborative commitment requires that the client and the clinician generally agree on procedures that are likely to be helpful. If the clinician has a strong commitment to interpretations of childhood conflicts or role playing or verbal therapy or play therapy or whatever, and this strikes the adolescent client as odd or uncomfortable or childish, progress is highly unlikely. If both the client and the clinician are committed to a process that makes sense to them, the second important element of collaborative commitment is that they both understand that their efforts need to be mutual. They are working together on the problem; the clinician is not there to fix the client. In fact, ideally, the balance is tipped toward the client being the primary problem solver with the collaborative support of the clinician.

Reinecke (1993) concludes from the research literature that "an active, collaborative approach may be useful in treating adolescents" (p. 402). He cites evidence in which adolescent clients expressed a consistent "desire for a therapist who could be a 'real person'—relaxed, caring, empathetic, active, and expressing affect spontaneously—yet who remains objective and insightful" (p. 402).

The Client Is the Problem Solver

It is obvious that the purpose of treatment is to find solutions for problems that are damaging the adolescent's life. It can be thought of as problem solving within the context of a good relationship. Many clinicians seem to think that it is their job to solve the adolescent's problems, but there are several reasons why it is most effective to help the adolescent solve his or her own problems.

Solving Problems and Getting Stronger The most obvious of these reasons is that helping a client become a problem solver carries two benefits: (1) immediate problems get solved, and (2) the client becomes stronger and more autonomous. All approaches to treatment focus on solving the client's problems, and nearly all say that one of their goals is increased independence and personal responsibility on the client's part. But there is a strange paradox here if the therapist is the primary problem solver. In a way, the therapist is saying, "You be independent because I am telling you to." The therapist's job is to empower the client. The most gratifying thing a clinician can hear from a client is, "I did this myself."

A Problem-Solving Focus Rather Than Deep Uncovering   Adolescents are far more comfortable with treatment structured as problem solving rather than as a deep uncovering of past traumas and the childhood causes of their troubles. Finding some way to communicate, "You will be solving your own problems; my job is to help you figure out ways to do that" provides a great benefit when working with adolescent clients. It makes sense to them as a way to proceed. It does not threaten their enormous need for autonomy, but it does support their enormous need not to be left alone to deal with their problems.

Treatment with adults often focuses on psychological insights, exploration of the past, and discussion of the psychological dynamics of both the client and others in the client's life. Adolescent clients, however, are generally less psychologically minded than adults and are often uncomfortable with these focuses. Weiner (1992) says:

> As for achieving deep insights and re-working previous experiences, adolescents typically have little patience with rehashing the vicissitudes of their earlier years. They are far too absorbed with the complexities and uncertainties of the present to spare much concern with matters they consider over and done with. Furthermore, their needs to view themselves as maturing, almost adult, almost self-sufficient individuals makes it distasteful and embarrassing for them to review their childish foibles of only a few years earlier. (p. 417)

This does not mean that adolescent clients never talk about their past, but when they do, the focus is usually problem solving oriented.

How Listening Contributes to Problem Solving

Much of the discussion in this chapter has focused on the way that deep listening helps to build and strengthen the personal bond between client and clinician. Listening, however, is also a clinician's most powerful tool for facilitating the client's problem solving. It does this in several ways.

First, as a good listener, the clinician will be articulating thoughts and feelings that the client has only implied and has not yet made explicit. If the client can feel, "Yes, that is what I meant, but I hadn't thought of that exactly that way. Now my own thought is clearer, and I can go further with it," then the process is empowering clearer thinking. We all have trouble articulating our thoughts and feelings at times, and having to explain them to someone else almost inevitably clarifies them. When a clinician articulates his or her understanding of the client's thoughts and feelings, the clarification process moves forward even more.

Second, the experience of having someone understand what you meant feels so good that it is a powerful reward both for talking and for thinking things through.

A third way that listening contributes to problem solving is more subtle and complex. It is based on the well-established principle that to reduce a fear of something, you must be exposed to the source of the fear and have nothing bad happen. One of the most important reasons that people do not think through their problems clearly is that many of the thoughts, feelings, and memories associated with the problem have become frightening. It is far more difficult to think or feel clearly about these particular frightening internal processes. When a client implies something, he or she is often trying to look at thoughts, feelings, and memories that carry a powerful emotional charge and are therefore difficult to make explicit. The clinician, by hearing this implicit meaning and putting it into words or somehow conveying that he or she has understood it, is helping the client stand in the face of something that is somewhat frightening. In doing so, and especially doing so in the context of a good relationship, the clinician helps to take the curse off the frightening thoughts, feelings, and memories. Now, together, the clinician and the client are bravely confronting thoughts, feelings, and memories that used to be mildly frightening. This process of confronting almost inevitably reduces the fear. The client will find it easier to think those thoughts and therefore will be free to move forward into even more difficult thoughts. To use the term from learning theory, the clinician is helping the client *extinguish* his or her fears related to problem solving—as it relates to specific issues and as it relates to problem solving in general.

Presenting Techniques as Tools
for the Client to Use

In the next chapter I describe techniques that you can use in treatment with adolescents. One problem with techniques is that they are often perceived by both clinicians and clients as procedures that the expert clinician applies to the treatment of clients. I return to this topic in more detail in chapter 3, but this is a good place to comment on how we can use techniques and still empower our clients as problem solvers. We can treat our techniques as information—as tools about which we know something and that we offer to the client to use or not to use, as he or she decides. We want to facilitate the client's own thinking, feeling, and taking action. If we clinicians make ourselves the experts, we deprive clients of the experience of solving the problems independently, and we will inevitably make errors in choices of goals. There is no reason, however, not to share our expertise on processes and principles with the client, as long as we honestly offer them as tools and not as (subtle?) manipulation. In fact, adolescents often receive the offering of techniques as a deeply empathic gesture and as a way that the clinician expresses interest and caring.

BEING THE INSTRUMENT THAT YOU ARE

Earlier I discussed the need to be forthright and genuine, but most clinicians struggle with how to do this while maintaining a professional identity. Sometimes clinicians, especially at the beginning of their careers, look for and cling to a set of techniques as *the* way to deliver treatment. In this chapter I have tried to focus on the principles behind what a clinician does, and I would like to set you free from the obligation to find the One True Way to be a clinician with adolescents. You need to find ways of being that are comfortable for you. You need to answer for yourself such questions as, How do I best connect with people? What techniques am I comfortable with?

I close this chapter by saying that if treatment is an interpersonal process, then each clinician needs to explore and understand how he or she is most effective in interpersonal relationships.

Recommended Reading

Spiegel, S. (1996). *An interpersonal approach to child and adolescent psychotherapy.* Northvale, NJ: Jason Aronson.

WORKING WITH THE INDIVIDUAL

CHAPTER 3

Techniques May Be Secondary, but They Are Important

In chapter 2 it was clear that much of the growth that happens during the treatment of an adolescent grows directly out of the complex process of being in a therapeutic relationship. The therapist's deep listening facilitates problem solving in many ways, and the experience of being in a good relationship is directly healing. Sometimes, clinicians get so caught up in their techniques that they see the relationship as little more than a necessary precursor that lays the groundwork for being able to apply their techniques. The relationship or therapeutic alliance, however, is often healing in and of itself. Having said that, I can now discuss many techniques that can enhance the process of treatment when used within the context of a good relationship.

In this chapter I focus on general techniques that can be used in most situations and on the principles that underlie those techniques. In a way, it is misleading to discuss highly specific techniques because the underlying principles can be applied in thousands of ways. If you understand those principles, you will be able to devise effective applications for the unique situations you will encounter in treatment. On the other hand, if you try to memorize a repertoire of specific techniques, you will be like a carpenter whose only tool is a hammer; you will treat everything as though it were a nail.

In the next chapter I explore special problems that arise in treatment and several kinds of direct interventions that clinicians can use. In later chapters I discuss specific treatment considerations for specific kinds of disorders and situations. If you understand the principles in chapters 2, 3, and 4, it will be clear to you how these principles might lead to different specific techniques—perhaps stricter setting of limits with some clients or a strong focus on emotional issues with others; some disorders call for more cognitive exploration, and other disorders require self-control anger management techniques.

THE ADOLESCENT'S NEED FOR STRUCTURE

Adult clients are usually comfortable with therapy that involves talking as its primary vehicle. Child clients often do best in play therapy, where they can use toys and other materials to supplement their verbal expressions. Adolescent clients, however, are too old to play with toys and often too young to be comfortable with a primarily verbal format. This means that working with adolescents requires a creative use of various kinds of structure, both to help the client feel more comfortable and to promote talking, self-exploration, and problem solving. These kinds of structure include the use of more questions, therapist self-disclosure, providing treatment in many different settings, and structured mutual activities, such as building models, playing pool, going for walks, meeting in a restaurant for lunch, or simply driving around listening to music and talking together. Research suggests that with adolescents "traditional long-term individual psychotherapy is less effective than briefer and more focused psychotherapeutic interventions" (Reinecke, 1993, p. 400). Throughout this book you will find many suggestions of the kinds of structure that are helpful in treating adolescents.

Setting up the Treatment Environment

An important part of the structure of treatment is the setting in which it takes place. If you were to meet an adult client who is a businessperson in an office that was slightly cluttered with art materials and in your casual clothes, you would probably lose credibility, and that credibility would be hard to regain. Similarly, the environment in which you first meet your adolescent client will have a significant impact on the client's first impression. The setting does make a difference.

Establishing a Comfortable Environment   You will probably see your adolescent clients in a wide variety of settings. If you do treatment in an activity group, for example, you might be in a room with craft supplies, books and magazines, a chalkboard, or other equipment designed to facilitate the group process. However, you may be working in an office most of the time. The appearance of and the equipment in your office will have a significant impact on your client's initial reaction to the treatment process. An effective strategy is to have a wide range of objects and materials available for the client to notice without their being so obvious that the client thinks using the materials is required. A good supply of paper, markers, and other art supplies should always be available. Hats, hand puppets, small stuffed animals, playing cards, and games that can be finished relatively quickly (*Monopoly* is a bad choice, normally) make good but subtle attention getters that may or may not be useful later as activities in treatment. It is important to have objects that appeal to a wide range of ages, because older clients sometimes will be put off by choices that seem too childish. One reason that your collection of materials should be visible but unobtrusive is that this implies that you see clients of many different ages and that you would not expect your client to be interested in, for example, hand puppets. This often provides an older adolescent client with the freedom to "jokingly" pick up a hand puppet and use it just for fun or sometimes as a means of expressing significant thoughts and feelings.

I often have my laptop computer sitting off to the side but obviously ready to use. There are many nonviolent, relatively simple but entertaining computer games that you and a client can play together while you also talk about other things. The computer seems to have a special appeal as relatively cool.

Designing your treatment area to be an interesting, comfortable setting serves several purposes. It can reduce your client's anxiety, help to establish you as an approachable and not-too-stuffy adult, and provide a wide variety of ways for your client to express thoughts and feelings.

The Therapist's Personal Appearance   The therapist's clothing and personal appearance have a significant impact on forming a connection with an adolescent client. The therapist needs to find a comfortable range somewhere between formal business attire and faddish teenage clothing. Adolescents who say, "My shrink is a suit" are probably expressing a resistance to the authority implied by highly formal clothing. On the other hand, when your clients talk to other adolescents about you (and they often will), you do not want them referring to you as a teenage wannabe. It is possible to dress in a way that seems casual and approachable to adolescents but that maintains a professional appearance. Obviously, your clothing and appearance will depend to some extent on the activities that you and your clients engage in. If you are going to shoot baskets, you should probably invest in a reasonably cool pair of basketball shoes.

Limits of Office-Based Practice   With adult clients it is most common for clients to visit the therapist's office and to spend 50 minutes talking. Relatively few adolescents are comfortable using this format for extended periods of time. If you limit your practice to office-based therapy, you will automatically limit the kinds of adolescent clients that you will see. There will be a powerful selection bias for a relatively narrow range of highly verbal clients.

A balance must be struck between the clinician's need for an efficient use of time and finding a setting that promotes therapy with the adolescent. One therapist I know has a small pool table in his office. Arranging your office to provide many activities helps to overcome some of the limits of office-based practice, but you also have to find a creative variety of settings and activities to get many of your clients comfortable enough to engage in treatment.

Principles of Brief Treatment

Much treatment that is offered to adolescents is relatively brief, for several reasons. Many adolescents are in volatile situations that provide only brief windows of opportunity for treatment; others resist long-term involvements as threats to their autonomy. For many adolescents long-term treatment does not make sense to them as a way to proceed; in their view, they have a problem, and they want that problem solved. In addition to reasons that are part of being an adolescent, however, external and economic forces also frequently demand that treatment be brief. Only a select group of families, for example, can afford extended individual treatment without outside help from insurance or social agencies. In recent years insurance companies and managed care organizations have tended to support briefer and briefer forms of treatment, largely for economic reasons. Whatever the causes for the need to offer brief treatment, the clinician should be familiar with the principles behind brief treatment.

Actually, all the techniques I have been discussing also apply to brief treatment, but they are used within a more structured and limited context. Swift (1993) describes three key principles that are fundamental to brief psychotherapy with adolescents.

It is no surprise that Swift's first principle is "to establish and maintain a therapeutic relationship" (p. 375). Swift notes that this is not an easy process with adolescents, primarily because of their need to separate from adults and build their own autonomy. This is "by no means an insurmountable obstacle, but the therapist needs to be aware of it" (p. 375).

Swift notes that the second key principle in brief psychotherapy is to find a specific focus for treatment. He means two things by this. Focus can mean that, even though the client's life includes a large number of problem areas, a treatment program centers around one or two of those areas. For example, the clinician might choose to concentrate on improving communication between an adolescent client and his or her mother. Because of limited resources and time, it may be necessary to give relatively little attention to communication with the client's father, academic performance, drug use, or any other possible problems. If it turns out that resources are available to broaden the focus of treatment, so much the better, but the strategy is that improving one specific area of the adolescent's functioning will have a positive effect on his or her life in general. Second, focus can also refer to a focal theme or issue in the client's life. Impulsiveness, low self-esteem, loneliness, and anger are examples of possible focal themes that might structure the focus of brief treatment. None of this means that only communication with the mother can be dealt with and only the focal theme can be discussed. Rather, the clinician is trying to focus treatment within the structure of a limited time period.

"The third principle of brief psychotherapy is to set modest, reasonable, and achievable goals" (Swift, 1993, p. 377). For example, the goal of empathic communication between mother and client, unconditional acceptance of each other, and constructive problem solving might be too ambitious and ultimately discouraging for brief therapy. If the client's focal theme is intense anger, significant reduction in hostility that results from a major personality change might also be more appropriate for longer-term treatment rather than brief therapy. Brief therapy is more likely to be successful and re-warding if its goals are more limited, such as reducing by half the frequency of yelling between a client and his mother and finding some strategy for the client to use to avoid violent outbursts.

ACTIVITIES

Probably the most obvious structural difference between treatment of adolescents and treatment of adults is that adolescents are far more likely to engage in the process if it is embedded in interesting activities.

Is This High Level Play Therapy?

Play therapy with young children serves the primary purposes of giving the child something entertaining to do while engaging in therapy and providing a means of expression at an age when ver-bal expression is more limited. Dolls, hand puppets, modeling clay, art supplies, and acting out scenes with toys all give the child a lan-guage to speak with. Adolescent clients also often need something entertaining to do, but this is more likely to be seen as "something to do while we talk." As we saw in chapter 2, however, well-chosen activities can also be a channel of communication for adolescents, through such things as music lyrics. I discuss a few such activities, but each clinician needs to be creative and thoughtful about choos-ing activities for individual adolescent clients. The principle is to provide a vehicle for making clients comfortable, engaging them in treatment, and giving them a way to express themselves—to talk, explore, and let themselves be known by you.

Activities That Establish Initial Comfort

Starting the treatment process is often terribly uncomfortable for adolescent clients, but activities can ease this transition. In chap-ter 2 I discussed ways that the clinician can help structure treat-ment for the adolescent by saying such things as, "Together we can figure out ways to improve things in your life that are not the way you would like them to be." For many adolescent clients the implicit expectation for them simply to start talking about their problems is daunting. Some clients, of course, do simply start talking and find this format for counseling perfectly comfortable. If, however, you sense uneasiness, awkwardness, or confusion about the process, it is usually helpful to broaden and normalize the process by saying something such as, "What I usually do when I'm working with someone is to talk about things, but that's not the only thing we can do. Sometimes it's easier to talk if we also have something else to do, like use any of the things here in the office or even build a model together or go for a walk" (or whatever activities you have available and with which you are comfortable).

There is a fine line to walk here. You are trying to establish that you and your client are engaged in an important and serious process but that you want him or her to be comfortable and not to be overwhelmed by the process. If you simply present the activities available as what you and the client will be doing together, most adolescents will see it as artificial and a bit silly, because "just playing" will not make sense to them as a reasonable treatment process.

Using Games

Board games, card games, and even computer games can also be useful ways to engage an adolescent client. There are, however, a number of issues to consider when choosing your games. No-brainer games such as the card game *War* or even *Crazy Eights* can give you something to do with your hands while you talk without introducing a large competitive element. If you choose chess or checkers or some other highly competitive board game, you must consider the implications of winning and losing. If you are much better at the game than your client, you will have to deal with the consequences of your client's always losing, or you will have to lose intentionally and risk the highly likely outcome that your client will see through you. Even if you and your client are evenly matched, one of you wins and one loses. It may be that this situation will provide you with opportunities to deal with your client's issues over frustration at losing, trust in you, and good sportsmanship, but those may or may not be the issues that you should be dealing with most in treatment. There is a risk that your choice of game will determine the focus of therapy.

If you use computer games as part of treatment, the impact of graphic violence must also be considered. One advantage of computer games is that some role-playing and adventure games provide a way for you and the client to cooperate in solving problems and achieving goals, such as outsmarting the wizard or building a city together in one of the simulation games (for example, *SimCity*).

There also are games that are specifically designed to facilitate self-exploration in the treatment of children and adolescents. For example, The Talking, Feeling, and Doing Game (1973, Creative Therapeutics, 155 Country Road, Cresskill, NJ 07626) is a board game that uses different kinds of activity cards that permit the participant to earn points to advance along the board. A player might draw a card, for example, that says, "Make believe that something is happening that's very frightening. Explain why it is frightening." Rather than requiring the player to act something out, other cards might ask evocative questions, such as, "Who's the luckiest person you know? Why did you choose this person?" Some of the cards are less pointedly psychological but still give players an opportunity to talk about themselves. For example, a card might ask, "What is your favorite smell?" A colleague of mine who uses this game says that she uses it only with groups of adolescents. However, she finds that using the game board introduces a competitive element that detracts from the therapeutic process; she believes that it is much more effective simply to use the cards to prompt activities and discussion.

For a game to be useful in treatment, it has to be presented to adolescent clients as something they can choose to do rather than as something that is being done to them. My colleague finds the game more acceptable to a group of adolescents than to individual clients. This also is my experience, although some therapists are successful with games in individual treatment. In individual treatment many adolescents react to such games as artificial, too obviously psychological, and uncomfortably intrusive. This often is expressed by calling the game stupid, perhaps directly to the clinician but, more likely, to other adolescents. In a group the intrusiveness of the game is diluted and is a more acceptable way to stimulate discussion among group members. My colleague reported one incident in which a client answered the question, "Who's the luckiest person you know?" by naming one of the other clients in the group and saying, "Because he has a mom and a dad who care about him." This comment stimulated meaningful interaction that probably would not have occurred otherwise. I think that the wisest course of action is to have a self-exploration game available in your office and to present it casually to test the waters with clients who might respond positively to it.

Drawing and Painting

We have seen that the well-equipped office should include paper, markers, and other art supplies. These are useful both as an activity to give you and the client something to do with your hands while you are talking and as a means for your client to express thoughts and feelings that might be more difficult to initiate simply with words. Drawing and painting are also often used as assessment tools. In the Draw a Person Test the clinician asks the client to draw a picture of a whole person. It should not be a stick figure or a cartoon figure, but beyond this the client is free to draw any kind of person. Some clinicians use this as a diagnostic tool and as the basis for making interpretations to the client. However, interpretation must be done with great caution, and, in fact, the evidence that exists for the reliability and validity of the Draw a Person Test is not convincing (Smith & Dumont, 1995). There is serious danger that the clinician will be inaccurate in making interpretations this way. However, the Draw a Person Test and any other drawing and painting can be useful stimuli for discussion during treatment.

Asking the adolescent to explain what the drawing or painting means, responding empathically to the explanation, and then even making shrewd but tentative guesses, which you check with the adolescent for accuracy, frequently bring difficult topics out into the open, making them available for future discussion. Occasionally, adolescent clients will bring in drawings or paintings that they have done outside treatment, and it is usually productive to ask penetrating and interested questions about what these drawings or paintings mean and how important they are to the client. Of course, you would follow up the questions with deep listening. If the client offers to give me such artwork, I accept it graciously and care for it well with the thought that the client and I may refer to this artwork sometime in the future. It is nearly always important to the client that I take good care of this artistic offering.

Kahn (1999) argues that art therapy is an especially useful medium for working with adolescents, no matter what other approaches the clinician uses in treatment. She says that art therapy is consistent with the adolescent's developmental tasks of becoming an individual and separating from the family. Art therapy provides the adolescent with personal control over the expression of thoughts and feelings, the opportunity for creativity, a pleasant experience, and media that permit the highly personal use of symbols and metaphors. "Adolescents live in the world of images; therefore they are comfortable with the therapy process utilized in images. Using images is additionally therapeutic in that it decreases the defenses, which typically slow traditional talk therapy. In nonverbal processes, counselors are not as likely to be drawn into the role of an authority figure" (Kahn, 1999, p. 292).

Kahn also has many practical suggestions for integrating art into treatment. "An art station should be equipped with some relatively fast media such as pastels, felt tip pens, and crayons. . . . In other situations, a counselor may specifically provide materials that will take longer to use and are more difficult to control. . . . Employing materials such as watercolors and clay generally allows (clients) greater artistic expression with more time to verbally process the experience" (p. 293).

Kahn divides art therapy into three general stages: entry, exploration, and taking action. During the exploration and taking action phases, she uses art directives, such as suggesting to the client, "Create a collage that depicts your understanding of why you're coming to counseling. . . . Make a collage that represents your family's communication. . . . Draw a bridge, representing where you are now and how you will be when counseling is completed; what are the obstacles in your way? What are the steps that need to be accomplished?" (p. 295). In each of these cases, the artwork is used as a vehicle for discussing and processing what the client is trying to communicate.

Food as a Vehicle

When I was discussing the Talking, Feeling, and Doing Game with my colleague (who has an excellent reputation as a clinician with adolescents), she laughingly said, "Then when all else fails, I give them candy." Behind her laughter, though, was an essential truth. The sharing of food is a powerful ritual in our culture, and breaking bread together is a source of bonding and giving each other comfort and spiritual nourishment. Using food as part of treatment does have some risks, but, done wisely, it can improve a client's mood, help build a personal bond, and make a client feel cared for.

If you are working in an office, it is a good idea to maintain a supply of drinks and snacks that are not junk food but are attractive to adolescents. You can introduce these snacks by taking one for yourself and offering one to your client; some clinicians like to make the snack a part of the starting ritual of each session. The sharing of food as an opening ritual is especially effective when working with adolescents in group treatment. Many of you will work in agencies or institutional settings with facilities for food preparation. Making pizza together, baking muffins, and cooking dinner often provide some of the richest opportunities for therapeutic moments. You and your client can talk when it feels right or you can busy yourselves with a mutually creative activity when the words just aren't there.

I sometimes take my adolescent clients to a restaurant for coffee or even for lunch. Even though we do not have the privacy of an office, these discussions over food are often productive and filled with more personal talk than what usually happens in an office setting. As helpful as this can be, though, it does raise some important issues about appropriate boundaries in treatment. I will return to the issue of boundaries and limits in treatment, but the fundamental principle is that the clinician remain just that—the clinician. The risk is that the relationship might become an ambiguous and confusing mixture of therapeutic relationship and friendship or other personal relationship. The clinician usually does not have to make a pointed issue out of this but should be sensitively aware of it as a potential problem.

Activities Must Be Clearly Structured as Part of Treatment

You should know that some clinicians would consider taking an adolescent client to lunch an inappropriate violation of boundaries, but there are many adolescents who will not benefit from nor participate in treatment confined to an office setting. They may well benefit from going to lunch, playing pool, walking in the park, or visiting the zoo if these activities are structured as part of treatment. The focus remains on the process of helping the client find new and better ways to live life, and it is not just "playing pool." The activity is a vehicle for the treatment process. The fundamental principle is that your client be clear that such activities are not friendship, casual companionship, or just for fun; they are part of treatment, and your relationship is still client/clinician.

In addition to making sure that the clinician's role always remains clear for the client, there is another risk in using lunch (or any activity outside the office) as a therapeutic activity. The clinician must protect him- or herself from the potential for accusations of inappropriate behavior. There is no absolute protection against this, but it is important that all your activities with a client outside the office be known to others. Meet your client in public places, document your meetings in your records, and be sure that appropriate other people are fully aware of when and where you are meeting with clients.

Vehicles as a Vehicle

For many adolescent clients, riding in a car is a remarkably fruitful environment for talking about personal issues. There are many situations in which clinicians who work with adolescents will be driving somewhere with the client. If you work for an agency or an institution, you may be driving clients to other appointments, for home visits, to community activities, to school, and so on. Riding in a car seems to create an atmosphere in which the official purpose is traveling from one place to another but where "we might as well be talking while we're here." Some other clinicians (Katz, personal communication, 1998) and I sometimes half jokingly say that we do car therapy. There are probably many reasons that riding in a car makes it easier for some adolescents to talk. Many, for example, find great comfort simply in riding around. It may make talking easier because both people are generally facing forward, perhaps lowering the intensity of the interaction. We also saw in chapter 2 that having music playing, either on the radio or on tape or CD, can provide a comforting background environment, or it can provide the structure and content for discussion when the lyrics are relevant.

Risks and Boundaries

In the previous section I discussed going to lunch or other activities with the client. This often involves a car ride. It may well be that the time in the car is as helpful as anything else the clinician is doing. I also need to repeat and emphasize the previous section's discussion of maintaining appropriate boundaries and protecting the clinician from damaging accusations. If you engage in car therapy, you will be more comfortable if you can account for all of your time in the car. The risks of being alone with a client are increasing, because the clinician could be accused of exploitative behavior. Activities outside the office can be powerful and effective, so it would be a significant loss just to abandon them, but you should protect yourself by formally informing someone when the activity begins and by making the activity as public as possible. It is also possible that such activities as car therapy would not be covered by insurance programs, and this might be an important consideration for you.

Helping the Adolescent Feel Known through Activities

In chapter 2 I said that one of the most healing things that a clinician can give to a client is the experience of being known accurately. Perhaps the most useful way to do this is through the deep listening that I discussed, but being engaged in activities also offers many opportunities to make an adolescent feel that "this person really knows me as I am." There will be hundreds of simple little moments that give this feeling. Even saying things such as, "You really like this, don't you?" when you see your client enjoying an activity or "You seem bored. Do you want to do something else?" have a cumulative effect in building your relationship. Even more powerful is the act of showing interest in your client's favorite activities.

Adolescent clients use many more languages than adult clients, and it is the clinician's job to be listening at every level for what the client is trying to say. We have seen how many activities provide opportunities for the client to talk, but the value of activities is also found in the way they help adolescent clients express themselves. Talking about favorite music, drawing, building models, baking pizza, playing games, and telling jokes can all make your client feel known, depending on how well you hear all these nonverbal languages.

THERAPEUTIC MOMENTS

In education there is much talk about teachable moments, in which students make dramatic advances in understanding. These moments probably do not come out of the blue; at other, less exciting moments the student is probably acquiring knowledge that will contribute to the teachable moment, but this just seems to be the laying of groundwork for the time when previous knowledge, motivation, emotional state, and focus all seem to come together in a flash of insight or in a qualitatively new level of understanding. It is almost as though the teacher slogs along for a long time, and then the moment just happens. Obviously, the slogging along for a long time was essential for the teachable moment to happen.

Treatment with adolescents often involves what we might call therapeutic moments. Something like this seems to happen in therapy with adults too, but it is more clearly a part of therapy with adolescents. With adults the process of self-exploration is fairly steady and issues are discussed with occasional experiences of increased clarity that stand out. With adolescent clients the process of growth seems less steady. As with the teacher, the clinician may feel treatment slogging along as groundwork is being laid. This groundwork consists of forming the therapeutic relationship, the client becoming comfortable with and learning how to talk about personal issues, and clarifying and articulating the content of the client's life. Laying this groundwork is itself therapeutic, but it is less exciting than the flashes of therapeutic moments. As clinicians, we need to draw two lessons from this. First, we need to understand the importance of being alert to therapeutic moments. Second, understanding this process can make us more patient with the slogging.

Learning to Recognize Therapeutic Moments

Much of the time that you spend with your adolescent client will be devoted to the kind of slow slogging that I have been talking about. Part of your job is to recognize the moments when something has touched your client in a deep way or when your client has something special to say to you that he or she is having difficulty putting into words. There are some cues that I can articulate here to help you recognize therapeutic moments, but most of your ability to do this will depend on your sensitivity to when your client is trying to say something that he or she really wants you to hear.

A clinician should be especially open to subtle, poignant emotion. Sometimes this will be signaled by misty eyes or an unusual thoughtful pause. Tone of voice might communicate anger, exasperation, sadness, or any other emotion. These moments are almost always important and should be acknowledged in some way, but the clinician has to walk a fine line between ignoring the meaning of the emotion and making too much out of it. If adolescents feel that an adult is making a big deal of their emotion, they often feel intruded upon and will be less likely to reveal emotion in the future. Often a comment such as, "You really don't like that do you?" or "Sounds like that bugs you" are just right to acknowledge the emotional meaning without intruding. Obviously, the clinician's response that will be just right depends entirely on what the client meant, the strength of the therapy relationship, and the intensity of the emotion.

But He's Not Working on His Issues!

Some people have a limited and stereotyped expectation of what qualifies as treatment of emotional problems. If the client is not discussing big feelings or working on his issues, it looks to these people as though no real work is being done. This expectation is based on the limited belief that treatment is primarily a clearly defined and obvious process of rational analysis, finding the causes of behavior, and establishing intellectual insight. This is a limited belief because, although there is a valid place in treatment for big feelings and working on issues and rational analysis, much progress in treatment is gradual and cumulative and quite ordinary seeming. This is especially true with adolescent clients, who are more likely to be taking important but small steps toward gradually becoming more confident or less aggressive or clearer about their own identities. Much of this happens while making pizza and just talking in the kitchen of a treatment facility or while drawing pictures or just going for a walk.

USING QUESTIONS TO GIVE STRUCTURE THAT HELPS THE ADOLESCENT

Asking questions is a more important part of treatment with adolescents than with adults. Questions can provide helpful structure, but they also can slow progress. The use of questions in therapy is a controversial topic. Brodsky and Lichtenstein (1999) have gone as far as to write a journal article called "Don't Ask Questions." They argue that therapy, especially therapy with unwilling clients, is impeded by the use of questions. Approaching a client with questions sets a tone of inquisition, intrusion, and information gathering. They argue that questions are typically used to help therapists cope with clients' silence and resistance and that questions implicitly structure therapy as a process of looking for the causes of behavior rather than as a process of problem solving and emotional growth. There is much truth to their arguments, especially as applied to therapy with adult clients. It is no accident that beginning therapists ask more questions than experienced ones do (Ornston, Cicchetti, Levine, & Fierman, 1968). For one thing, experienced therapists can live through silences and even see them as constructive. For another, experienced therapists are more skillful at presenting a thought as a statement rather than as a question.

With adolescent clients some kinds of questions do impede therapy, but some kinds of questions facilitate the process in ways that seem unique to adolescent clients. The general principle is that harmful questions focus on evidence gathering: asking the client various versions of, "Why did you do that?"; probing beyond areas that the client is comfortable with; and asking questions that the adolescent perceives as stupid because they reveal a lack of understanding of something that should be obvious. The kinds of questions that facilitate treatment with adolescents include the empathic questions that I discussed previously, questions that give permission to talk but do not intrude, questions that help the adolescent explore what he or she is thinking and talking about, and questions that show interest.

We need to understand effective and ineffective questions extremely well to work with adolescent clients because they seem to need the structure that questions can provide more than adult clients do, but they are painfully sensitive to questions that intrude on their autonomy. I have often said that adolescent clients are less psychologically minded than adult clients; this also applies to their understanding of what one does in treatment. Adult clients are far more likely to expect that they will do most of the talking during treatment. Adolescent clients are more likely to sit blankly and expect the clinician to ask questions.

Questions Are Easy

Brodsky and Lichtenstein (1999) are probably correct when they say that a primary function of using questions is to help the therapist cope. Questions are often an easy way to mask our own confusion and inability to think of what to say and to focus the attention back on the other person. We depend on questions to get responses from other people, to fill in awkward silences, to gather information, and to solve problems. Questions are easy to depend on because they demand a response, and so we use them a lot. When the other person is talking to us, asking a question implies that we want more information, but it may fail to communicate that we have understood the information we have just received. Adolescent clients often require more questions, but you must be clear about the impact of the kind of questions you ask.

Empathic Questions Revisited

I have already discussed the most powerful kind of question you can use. Empathic questions prove that you have understood what the other person was trying to say. Sometimes they achieve this by referring to an emotion that the clinician is sure the client was implying in his or her communication. The clinician might use an empathic question instead of a statement to soften the intensity of the response, to make it easier for the client to reject the response if it feels too strong or inaccurate, or to add a tentativeness if the clinician is not quite sure he or she has understood correctly. In addition to helping to name implicit feelings and meanings, the clinician can use empathic questions to prove that he or she understood the factual content of what the client said. For example, you might have a client who said, "If you have more than ten absences, the principal talks to you." You could ask a factual question such as, "What would he do to you?" This question did not explicitly express an understanding of what the client said, but you could have asked the question only if you did understand. Actually, your question also proved that you understood the client's implicit message that his statement applied to his own situation, even though he stated it somewhat generically.

Questions That Give Permission to Talk but Do Not Intrude

I have discussed how empathic questions can give the client emotional permission to talk about topics that have been strongly implied but that the client is having difficulty pursuing. With adolescents it is sometimes helpful to go beyond what they are communicating, if you have a pretty good idea that there is a topic they need and want to talk about. This obviously requires a delicate sensitivity and gradual approach to the topic in order not to be perceived as intrusive and controlling. If you know a client well, for example, and have good reason to believe that he or she is the victim of abuse that has never been spoken of, you might ask questions about topics that are distant enough so as not to be threatening but that put words on the table about the general topic of abuse.

Questions That Explore

Schubert (1977) describes several kinds of questions therapists ask and argues that only one of them is really helpful. *Genuine questions* ask for the client's personal view of an event or experience and can be answered only by the client. The quality that makes genuine questions helpful is that they are offered in the spirit of "I am really trying to understand this with you" or "I would like to know how it is for you" or "I want to know your story." The risk is that the clinician will seem to ask genuine questions that are really *manipulative questions*. Manipulative questions are designed to lead the other person to a particular conclusion chosen by the questioner. The questioner is not interested in the answer but in getting the other person to admit he or she is wrong.

Questions that help the client explore seem to be more useful with adolescent clients than with adult clients, largely because adolescents are less comfortable with initiating discussion. The most effective pattern is to mix together exploring questions and responses that show deep understanding of the answers. A string of questions is far less effective than asking a question and then responding to your client's answer by articulating what the answer implies in a way that makes it clear that you got the point.

Questions That Show Interest

Another kind of question that can be helpful is the question that demonstrates interest in topics in which the client is interested. It serves several purposes to ask your client to educate you about fishing, rap music, current fashion, football, or whatever he or she is fascinated by. Your interest will help to build a bond between you, it will reward your client for talking to you and for talking in general, and it will teach you many things you never knew and probably should know about the world of adolescents. One of my adolescent clients was extremely withdrawn and would say virtually nothing to anyone at the treatment facility where he was periodically hospitalized. He was, however, fascinated with the stock market, and he and I talked comfortably for hours while I asked questions and he educated me about the world of finance. These discussions formed the basis for his successful recovery.

Problems with Evidence-Gathering Questions

Adolescent clients are especially put off by Sherlock Holmes therapy. The therapist sets out looking for the facts, asking lots of evidence-gathering questions. The most destructive of these questions usually involve the word *why*. Some clinicians love to focus on a search for the causes of behavior, especially causes that force the adolescent to explain him- or herself. This question asking, especially in the first interview, creates a powerful set for the client. The client is learning how to engage in therapy and how therapy works by the example set by the therapist in this early encounter; it is not reasonable for the therapist to expect to ask a lot of questions and have the client suddenly start self-exploration. Even worse, most adolescents perceive this evidence gathering as an intrusive, controlling, and threatening attempt by an adult to fix them in ways they may not want to be fixed.

INTERPRETATIONS

Probably the most common stereotype of a clinician is of a person who gives interpretations, in the sense that he or she tells clients what is wrong with them, what the real and hidden meaning is of what they have said, and what they should do about their lives. Sometimes it is effective to give advice and to offer opinions to your adolescent client, as I discuss in many places in this book, but there probably is no faster way to lose an adolescent client than to interpret his or her behavior and thoughts as an expert.

Weiner (1992) says that "efforts in psychotherapy to penetrate an adolescent's defensive style tend to be unproductive, and interpretations designed to strip away whatever defenses can be found often have the counterproductive effect of mobilizing an adolescent's anxiety and attenuating his or her engagement in the treatment" (p. 417). The phrase "attenuating his or her engagement in the treatment" is a politely worded way to say that you will drive your client out of therapy with most traditional interpretations. For example, one 16-year-old client was accompanied by her social worker at what was supposed to be her first therapy session with another clinician. As the girl entered the office, her toe caught on the edge of a throw rug and she stumbled momentarily. The new clinician said, "You don't have to do that here in order to get attention." This kind of interpretation is often called a transference interpretation because it analyzes and explains aspects of the relationship between the client and the clinician. Mohr (1995) reviewed 46 studies of factors that contribute to the destructive effects of some therapists and concluded that several therapist behaviors stood out as destructive. Not surprisingly, these factors included a lack of empathy, negative feelings the therapist held for the client, and arguing with clients, but, of greater interest to us, they also included a high concentration of transference interpretations. The clinician's "cleverness" in telling the girl the "real meaning" of her stumble doomed any chance of forming a therapeutic alliance. This is not an unusual example, unfortunately. Many clinicians set themselves up as clever psychologizers rather than as facilitators of the client's own problem solving and growth.

Weiner (1992) states the case strongly when he says:

> All interpretations are implicitly critical, and every interpretation implies that the person is thinking, feeling, or doing something that is foolish or unwarranted. Consequently, repetitive interpretations of the coping behaviors of adolescent patients are likely to induce a self-consciousness that constrains them from the normal adolescent business of experimenting and also leads them to regard the therapist as a picky, hostile, disapproving person who is pessimistic about their future. A therapist who focuses extensively on irrational and unconscious motives for an adolescent's behavior risks communicating to the young patient, "I don't think much of you" or "I don't see much hope for you," either of which can undermine the adolescent's expectations that something good might come out of the treatment relationship. (pp. 416–417)

The Therapist as an Educated Guesser

The clinician can find ways to offer opinions, advice, and new understanding that the client is not aware of. The principle is that these are all offered as part of a mutual problem-solving process rather than as expert pronouncements. With adolescent clients Katz (1998) says that he sees himself as an "educated guesser. I know several reasons why something occurs, and I would like to see if any of them fit, or if the patient has a better suggestion. We work together" (p. 98). Katz often uses the term *educated guesser* with his clients because the term makes sense to adolescents. They can let him into their process without fear that he "thinks himself so wonderful that everyone will immediately want to work with him" (p. 98). If the clinician is just an educated guesser, he or she can offer suggestions, possible explanations, and other responses that are all very much like interpretations but do not threaten the client's autonomy. By this point it should go without saying that even educated guesses are effective only within the context of a good relationship. In chapter 2 I quoted an adolescent client as saying how important it was to have trust between the clinician and the client because "that way they don't seem so critical. . . . It's more like they're giving advice."

A good way to close these two chapters on working with the individual is with another statement from this client. "It's a trust thing." Techniques are important, but they are useless without the client's involvement (Bohart & Tallman, 1999), and the client must trust the clinician to become involved.

Recommended Reading

Riley, S. (2001). *Group process made visible: Group art therapy.* Philadelphia, PA: Brunner-Routledge.

Weiner, I. B. (1992). *Psychological disturbance in adolescence* (2d ed.). New York: Wiley.

4 CHAPTER TREATMENT ISSUES AND INTERVENTIONS

In some ways this chapter is an extension of chapter 3, because I continue to discuss techniques, but the focus moves on to handling difficult issues. In addition, I try to give a blend of theoretical principles and practical advice about how to handle special situations and how to use behavioral and cognitive behavioral interventions.

DIFFICULT ISSUES IN TREATMENT

Working with adolescents often involves some complicated dilemmas for the clinician. I cannot prepare you for all of these (which is why I hope you always have someone to consult, such as a colleague or supervisor), but there are several difficult issues that arise so frequently in working with adolescents that some practical advice is worth considering.

Missed Sessions and Lateness

Adolescent clients are significantly more likely than adult clients to miss sessions and to be late for sessions. My advice on how to handle missed sessions with adolescents is complicated, because so much depends on the consequences of how you handle the situation. With adult clients the issue is usually less complex, and you can have a few general policies, such as clients pay for sessions unless they give you 24 hours' notice or have a compelling reason. With adolescents, however, having a few general policies that you consistently enforce can easily lead to early termination with a large number of your clients. The danger is that the issue of missed sessions can become the focus of treatment and, even if this does not end treatment, it comes to dominate your time together, distracting you and your client from other issues. It may be, of course, that an important lesson your client must deal with is that of responsibility and consistency, and the missed sessions can provide an opportunity to talk about these issues. In addition, your time is a valuable and scarce commodity, and missed sessions can easily waste a lot of it.

It is unrealistic and not therapeutic to be completely permissive about missed sessions; on the other hand, focusing too much on missed sessions in a judgmental way can damage your relationship. However you decide to deal with missed sessions, for your own benefit it is usually wise to anticipate that you will have at least some missed sessions, and you should plan to have alternative ways to productively use the time that otherwise might be wasted. I try to have with me reading or some other activity that I need or want to do. This is only for the protection of the clinician's productive use of time. It should not provide the context to communicate to the client, "It's OK if you skip sessions, because it doesn't cost me anything; I always have other work to do." When you discuss missed sessions with your client, it may be useful to mention that you were able to use the time productively but that missed sessions are a problem that needs to be dealt with. This takes the focus away from "Look how much you cost me" and puts it on "Responsible behavior is an important thing to learn."

Silences

Dealing with silences is another aspect of counseling and therapy that is different with adolescent as opposed to adult clients. In therapy with adult clients periods of silence are usually a lot harder on beginning therapists than they are on clients. When I was in graduate school, another student and I were audiotaping role-played therapy, and he wanted to shut off the tape recorder during silences so as not to waste tape. The tape wasn't being wasted, of course, but there was something so nerve-racking about all that unfilled time that he had to do something to stop the process.

Our culture seems to teach us to hate silence, and clinicians are often tempted to fill all silences, either with their own chatter or with questions that get the client talking. As we have seen in previous chapters, questions can be helpful, but it is probably not a coincidence that beginning therapists ask more questions than experienced ones do (Ornston, Cicchetti, Levine, & Fierman, 1968). The important lesson is to learn how to listen to silences for what they mean to the client rather than in terms of the therapist's need. Sometimes the client is using the silence to think about or to explore or to assimilate something, and your need to fill that silence with chatter interferes with these processes. On the other hand, sometimes the client is acutely aware of the silence and is embarrassed and awkward about not having something to say. In the first case the helpful clinician would remain silently attuned while the client is using the silence. In the second case the most helpful thing to do is probably break the silence with some kind of understanding of how difficult it is, perhaps saying, "It's hard to get things into words, I guess" or "I can tell it's hard to get going. I suppose it could be just not knowing where to start or going blank or something like that." The clinician could say, "Would it help if I asked you some questions?" Or the most helpful thing might simply be to start asking questions that make it easier for the client to talk. The critical issue, obviously, is to have a clear sense of what the silence means to your client.

My experience has been that silences are more painful for adolescent clients than for adult clients. Adolescents are less likely to be using the silence to work something through. In previous chapters I discussed this same issue in the context of saying that adolescent clients need more structure. They tend to be less psychologically minded than adult clients and find silences difficult. They are more likely to feel understood when the clinician asks questions that reflect a sensitive knowledge of what is important to the client. In a funny way this is often a relief to the clinician, especially the beginning clinician. It is easier to ask questions than it is to communicate other kinds of deep understanding. I mention this only to sensitize you to the potential risk of becoming dependent on asking questions as your primary clinical tool.

Another caution about my saying that adolescent clients need more questions is that, obviously, this is not always true. Your job is still to listen sensitively for what the silence means to your individual client. Sometimes adolescents really do need to sit quietly in the presence of someone who understands and accepts them.

Sometimes adolescents use periods of silence productively to think things through. Sometimes you will have a client who is terribly upset but who cannot stand to talk about it. Every silence has its own meaning, and the skillful clinician is open to the unique meaning.

Reacting to Denial and Resistance

Both denial and resistance have two different meanings. Sometimes denial refers to serious self-deception in which the person misperceives his or her personal reality, and resistance can refer to another kind of self-deception in which the clinician tries to help the client understand something but the client cannot grasp it because it is emotionally threatening. These kinds of denial and resistance are defenses against anxiety and are the kinds of problems we can help clients with through therapy.

Dealing with adolescents, however, often involves a kind of conscious denial and resistance that could be characterized as defiant and uncooperative. Some adolescents are masters at infuriating adults by being defiant, dismissive, and condescending. It is difficult not to be drawn in by this kind of behavior and not to take it personally. Many times in your life as a clinician with adolescents you will have to respond to open rejection of what you do and say in such a way that you neither permissively let yourself be verbally abused nor respond angrily. It is the firm and caring or strong and helpful combination of qualities that seems necessary to help the mature clinician respond with good humor while maintaining his or her position. Sometimes, of course, you will have to set limits on clients' behavior, and I discuss this more later in the book.

Parental Contact

The relationship between you and the parent or parents of your adolescent client will range from relatively straightforward to extremely complicated and distressing. Parents often are threatened by the process of therapy and the knowledge that their adolescent has a special relationship with another adult, a relationship that is often perceived as designed to correct errors that the parents have made raising their child. The threat is compounded by the privacy of the treatment relationship, and it is almost inevitable that parents will wonder what is being said during sessions. Actually, they probably do more than wonder; they worry about what is being said.

Your relationship with parents is complicated by the fact that in most cases they still have legal responsibility for and control of their child. It requires delicate skill to help parents feel well treated and involved in the process (or at least not badly treated and excluded from the process) while earning your adolescent client's trust and the knowledge that you are his or her agent. Parents often do have the power to withdraw an adolescent client from treatment, but rather than just responding to this implicit threat to treatment, the clinician will find it helpful to enlist the parents' support of treatment.

There are several helpful ways that you can reassure parents that you are not their enemy and that you have some understanding of their position while gaining their support for the need for the treatment relationship to be special and confidential. One difficult situation that illustrates some general principles of how this can be done is when a parent phones you and says something such as, "There's something I have to tell you about John, but I don't want you to tell him that I told you." This situation is a minefield in which you risk betraying your client, offending the parent, or both. One helpful way to handle this situation is to quickly say something such as, "Can I stop you for a minute? There's something I need to say before you tell me. This is pretty complicated, and I can tell that you are concerned. It's important to me that my relationship with John be based on trust, as I'm sure you are aware." When the trust issue is presented in this way, most parents respond with some kind of agreement and understanding about the importance of trust. But there still is more that you need to say to the parent. I would add something like, "I have told John that I will discuss with him any conversations I have had about him with other people. I really need not to have secrets from him as part of our agreement." In essence, you have now warned the parent that he or she can say anything, but it should be said with the knowledge that it will be discussed with the client.

It would be naive to think that these few sentences will take care of all situations in which a parent phones you. Sometimes at this point the parent will add, "But you don't understand. This is something that you must know about, and I'm sure that John is not going to tell you. But if he knows I told you, he will be absolutely furious and will probably run away again." This puts you in a terrible dilemma. You are probably being manipulated and sabotaged, but there really may be something compelling that you need to know. It is almost always the wiser course, however, to find some way to protect the integrity of your relationship with your client. You must use discretion in how you present the nature of the parent's phone call to your client, but the important thing is that you have given yourself the freedom to determine what discretion means by warning the parent ahead of time that you must feel free to share what has been said with your client.

None of this means that parents should be excluded from the treatment process. In fact, parents often can and should be included as part of the treatment process, as I discuss in several other places in this book. The fundamental principle is to keep clear about whose agent you are and to help your clients know that you are on their side psychologically.

Giving Advice

Giving advice to adolescent clients is a tricky business. We often have information about how the world works that the client seems not to have, and it seems foolish and almost cruel not to share this information; we could save the young person so much grief from learning things the hard way. On the other hand, our primary goal is to strengthen our clients by facilitating their own problem solving and learning, and sometimes learning things the hard way provides deep understanding and strength.

There clearly are times when giving advice is the most helpful thing to do. Before I discuss that, however, I want to examine the potential risks of giving advice to young clients. I want to dwell on this a bit, because the urge to give advice is so overwhelming for most of us that we practically have to bite our tongues when a young person comes to us with a problem.

The biggest risk in giving advice probably is that virtually all adults give advice to adolescents frequently, and it usually arouses angry defensiveness. There are many reasons for this, but one of the most obvious is that the way most advice is given carries with it the implication of both judgment and control. If you want to avoid being lumped in with all these other adults, you must find a way to give advice that does not imply judgment and control. Another risk is implied: Giving advice can take away from the client an opportunity to solve a problem or find information independently. Finally, I promise you that some of the advice you give will simply be wrong, and this has many consequences. If your client compliantly follows your incorrect advice, you could easily make a situation worse. Poor advice also undermines your clients' trust in you. We really do need to be humble about how much we know about how another person should live his or her life. All our advice is filtered through our own needs, distortions, and unique experience, and it is based on our incomplete knowledge of the client's experience. As you know from previous chapters, we have powerful alternatives to giving advice, alternatives that help the young person solve his or her own problems.

When, then, is advice useful? Two general principles guide my answer to this question. First, if the clinician has important information that the young client is unlikely to discover for him- or herself, it is probably useful to share that information. Done sensitively, this advice can be delivered in a way that does not arouse defensiveness. In fact, it can be perceived by the young client as an expression of concerned helpfulness. You might say, "It sounds like you're having trouble with. . . . One thing that has worked for a lot of people is. . . . I don't know how that sounds to you or if you'd like to know more about it." Second, if your client is about to do something that will have severe consequences, giving advice is clearly justified, even if it means taking some control of the process. The problem here, obviously, is in defining severe consequences.

Confidentiality

The promise of confidentiality is fundamental to counseling and therapy. It frees the client to face thoughts and feelings that he or she couldn't otherwise face, because the client comes to trust the therapist's acceptance. The client doesn't have to worry about who else might hear these things and judge them. The kind of confidentiality you can promise to an adolescent client, however, is more limited than the confidentiality typical of treatment with adult clients. Because few of your clients will be old enough to be legally responsible for themselves, other adults will have some legal right to information about the therapy process. In a previous section I discussed ways to talk with parents to enlist their cooperation in valuing the need for confidentiality, but you probably cannot promise an adolescent complete confidentiality.

In any case, confidentiality always has limits, and these limits must be made clear to your client. There are, however, ways to word what you say to your client that honestly present the limits of confidentiality while minimizing the threat to the adolescent's trust of you and the process. I like to say something such as, "The things that you and I talk about are private between us, with a few exceptions. It's important to me that I explain those exceptions to you so you know where you and I stand and so you know what you can trust me with. The main thing is that I don't want to have secrets from you, so if I ever do have to talk with somebody about what we've talked about, I will try to discuss it with you ahead of time, and if I can't do that, I will tell you later what we talked about. For example, if your parents phone me, I will explain to them how important trust is between us, and I will say that I need to feel free to discuss with you whatever they talk to me about." This much is probably a lot to say to an adolescent client all at once, and I would probably get some reaction from my client or talk about something else for a little while before I explain the limits of confidentiality.

One limit on confidentiality is that professional considerations may require you to consult with another clinician about the course of therapy or about concerns you have, especially if you are working in an interdisciplinary treatment setting. You might say to a client, "Sometimes I will need to talk with another worker here, but I will let you know when that happens and whatever we say is still confidential within the staff."

Wording I have found helpful for other limits includes "I need to tell you that I can be subpoenaed to testify in court. That almost never happens, but you do need to know about it when you decide to tell me stuff." Another useful statement is a variation on, "Everything we talk about is private between us, but there are a couple of things that the law requires me to report. If I know about abuse of a child that has not been reported to a social agency, I am required to report that, and if a person was about to do something extremely dangerous to himself or somebody else, I would have to do what I could to prevent that."

Said all at once, this much talk about limits on confidentiality probably would seriously inhibit an adolescent, so I am not likely to present all of this in one long speech. I would intersperse it among other kinds of talk, especially talk in which my client feels understood and accepted. It also helps to present these limits in a straightforward, unapologetic tone that implies, "I'm sure it makes sense that of course these are reasonable limits." You wouldn't say this, of course, but you do imply it. Actually, these *are* reasonable limits, and most adolescent clients will recognize and accept that and will react positively to the trustworthiness implied in your being straightforward about them.

Inappropriate Boundaries

The relationship between a clinician and an adolescent client is special and unique. Nowhere else in the world are two people so focused on the emotional growth of one of them. You provide your client with remarkably attentive listening, intensely worked at under-standing, unusually dependable respect and acceptance, and the freedom to deal with all kinds of thoughts and feelings. Because these experiences are powerful, they must be provided within clear boundaries. Violating these boundaries can lead to terrible confu-sion for your client and can even do damage to your client, to you, and to other people. The fundamental principle that you must never forget is that you are the client's *clinician.* You are not a parent; you are not a substitute parent; you are not a friend; and you are not the savior of the person's life. As a client's clinician, you can provide a wonderful relationship and many things the person may not have elsewhere in life, but to be helpful, you need to provide this within a limited relationship.

The key difference between a clinical relationship and other re-lationships is that the clinician temporarily sets aside his or her needs in the service of what the client needs. In virtually all other relationships both people have needs that must be met. If the cli-nician needs to be loved by the client or needs to be seen as a sav-ior or hero or is trying to get other needs met through the relation-ship with the adolescent, the stage is set for trouble.

One primary function of boundaries and limits is to permit the therapist to function more fully within treatment. You provide your client with a remarkable intensity of understanding and acceptance that you could not maintain continuously. Knowing that the rela-tionship is limited sets you free to give more fully in the treatment process. There is no limit on what might be discussed in therapy, but, for example, the client is prohibited from harming you physi-cally. This knowledge frees both the therapist and the client to deal openly with feelings and thoughts of hostility toward the therapist. At the extreme, if a treatment session could last anywhere from 1 hour to 7 hours and if the adolescent were free to call you at any time to talk as long as he or she wanted to, you would have to pace yourself differently than if you know how much is going to be asked of you. Setting limits frees you to give more fully in the session.

Clear boundaries and limits also protect your client in several important ways. I have already mentioned that clear limits give the client freedom to discuss many difficult issues with the safety of knowing that the discussion is prohibited from leading to certain behaviors. Another way that the clinician's clear boundaries protect the client is important: If you somehow imply that your relationship is more than it really is, you are setting up your adolescent client to feel hurt and betrayed. You will be making promises that you cannot keep, and you will do damage. Finally, clear boundaries protect the client because they help prevent burnout in the clinician. Burnout is dangerous in many professions, but it is probably most dangerous in the helping professions. The risk is that clinicians who have trouble setting boundaries give more and more of themselves, trying to be helpful, until they are under so much stress from being overextended that they collapse and withdraw from their clients. "Collapse and withdraw" can mean many different things, but it frequently includes sudden, inexplicable, and horribly confusing coldness on the clinician's part.

Finally, I have to mention inappropriate boundaries in which a small percentage of clinicians use the treatment relationship to meet their own needs. These needs can range from a desire to be loved and admired to sexual gratification. Probably the most destructive thing that a clinician can do is exploit an adolescent client for his or her own needs.

Setting Limits and Using Direct Interventions

As a clinician working with adolescents, you will be in different roles at different times. In all cases it will be important to maintain appropriate limits in your relationships with clients, but sometimes those limits go beyond simply establishing a helpful structure for treatment and become consequences for the client's behavior. If your role involves only a therapeutic relationship that does not go beyond the walls of your office, you will seldom have to deliver consequences. There are many advantages to this, because delivering consequences complicates your relationship and in some ways inevitably interferes with the process of self-exploration and problem solving. Often, however, your role will be more complicated and will involve relationship formation, talking and listening, problem solving, intervening in the young person's environment, and delivering reasonable consequences for behavior. This complex role is in many ways the more difficult one to fill. However, it also has some advantages. Done well, filling this role in a young person's life can provide helpful corrective experiences that may undo damage done by other relationships.

Earning the Right to Deliver Consequences and Setting Limits without Judgment   Most clinicians at some time will be required to deliver consequences for behavior or to set limits on behavior. It takes great skill to do this without weakening the relationship with your client, because your young client will feel judged, but there are two important things you can do to avoid damaging the relationship. First, you should build a foundation for your relationship by repeatedly making your client feel understood and accepted as a person. You earn the right to deliver consequences and set limits by first laying this foundation. Second, when you do deliver consequences and set limits, you do it by focusing on behaviors and the natural consequences of behaviors rather than on the personal characteristics of your client. This may seem obvious, but it is discouraging to observe how many clinicians use such phrases as, "Your problem is your attitude" or "You are so self-centered that it will be difficult for you to have good relationships." Adults use these types of phrases with young people so often and so naturally that it is often difficult to see the subtle damage that they do. "Your attitude" and "self-centered" are such all-encompassing personal characteristics and are so difficult to change that they almost always arouse resistance and defensiveness. It is far better to say some version of, "When you do this, that happens." This names a specific behavior or set of behaviors (which can be changed), and it names the natural consequences of those behaviors.

A phrase that many people find helpful is *natural consequences* (or *reasonable consequences*). If consequences are delivered and limits are set in the context of their being natural consequences of behavior, then much of the judgment that the client perceives as, "You are bad or flawed or weak" is removed.

Probably more important, thinking of consequences and limits as natural consequences helps remove some of the implication of punishment. Discipline and limits are an essential part of dealing with a young person, but discipline and limits are dramatically different from punishments.

Preventing Disasters   Some of the principles I have discussed in the section on giving advice also apply to initiating direct interventions in the client's life. It is generally inconsistent with what I have been saying to view the clinician's role as taking direct action in changing the client's life circumstances as a therapeutic tool. In most cases the goal is to help the client solve problems and take the actions that will improve his or her life. Sometimes, however, direct intervention is necessary.

The most obvious of these circumstances is an emergency situation in which your client is at risk or is in immediate danger of harming him- or herself or another person. In addition to obvious emergencies, some situations will call for difficult decisions about your role in your client's life. If you are considering directly intervening in your client's life, it is almost always essential that you consult a colleague or supervisor in making your decision. There are consequences for directly intervening in a situation, and the need to intervene must be weighed against these consequences. Once you have intervened in your client's life, you have changed your role with your client. Instead of being the person who facilitates the client's own problem solving, you might become a person who can be useful in getting things for the client or a person who will take over control of things from the client.

Involuntary Clients

If you see adult clients, in most cases they are people who have chosen to seek your help and probably even pay for it. However, a large number of adolescent clients—maybe even most of them—enter treatment because somebody else wants them to. There is nothing you can do to force an adolescent to enter into the treatment process. You could conceivably force your client to go through the motions of treatment by attending sessions and even possibly completing therapeutic homework assignments you might give. But this is not the same as the client's being involved in the process. Bohart and Tallman (1999) argue persuasively that the best predictor of success in therapy is whether or not the client is involved in the process. We need to think in terms of what might help this happen with involuntary clients.

What's in This for Me?   In general, people do what they are reinforced for doing. I often find it helpful to think in these terms when I am first talking to an involuntary client. I try to think, from the client's perspective, what he or she has to gain from entering into the treatment process. There are often many reasons we give to adolescents for why they should cooperate with us, reasons that do not really makes sense from the adolescent's point of view: "You need help," "The court sent you," "You're getting in trouble at school," "You have a drug problem," "You need to control your anger." Whatever the adolescent answers about these reasons, he or she is often thinking, "So what?" "That's not my problem" or "Tough."

You might want to refer back to the discussion of the importance of the early sessions in therapy with adolescents—and even the importance of the first few minutes of contact. Your initial contact with the client who doesn't want to be there and is ready to do battle is especially important. You have a few minutes to hook your client by giving him or her a reason to trust you as an individual and a reason to engage in the process. The most effective way to establish yourself as someone worth talking to is to demonstrate quickly that you can understand your client's experience and that you are on the client's side in terms of wanting good things for the client. As I said in chapter 2, much of this is accomplished by saying such things as, "I know you don't really want to be here, and if I were in your shoes, I would be suspicious and skeptical of somebody like me." Some version of this statement is often useful in making your initial contact. In addition to this general kind of understanding, of course, you should be listening intently for some unique meaning that your client is implying about his or her current feelings and experiences and wishes. Putting that understanding into words will be especially powerful in engaging your adolescent client, because he or she will be sure that you are not going to listen and will be surprised and put at ease and intrigued by an adult who gets it.

Even if you are deeply understanding and easy to talk to, you will probably still be perceived as an agent of the system, of parents, or even of adults in general. At some level your involuntary client expects adults to have an agenda that primarily involves doing something *to* the adolescent. It is usually helpful to acknowledge this suspicion and to talk in terms of what the client has to gain from the process, as the client perceives "gain." You might say something to the effect of, "My guess is that you have basically been sent to therapy because other people want you fixed somehow. I'm also guessing that you don't really have a clue what to expect from me and from what we're supposed to be doing. OK, let me talk for a minute or two about how I see what we're supposed to be doing. My understanding is that anger and violence have gotten you in enough trouble that you have been charged with a legal offense, and people want you to find some way to control your anger. Well, that's almost certainly something we should think about working on, but I really think in broader terms. What I want to do in our work together is to find ways to make your life better, whatever 'better' means to you. And I don't know what that is ahead of time. I'm not even sure what you would say if I asked you what would make your life better, but I think I'm pretty good at helping kids figure out ways to improve their lives." This is a pretty long speech for a therapist to be making, especially early in treatment, and I might get these thoughts across over the course of several minutes, stopping to listen and to make my client feel understood every chance I got.

Give Me Three Sessions   Almost all adolescents have an issue with establishing their autonomy and are sensitive to what they perceive as control by adults. One way to diminish the intensity of this barrier between you and your involuntary client is to talk in terms of a brief, limited, initial time contract between you. After you have established a good contact with the client and talked about how your goals are to help him or her find ways to improve life, it can be helpful to say something such as, "Why don't we try this for three sessions, and if you don't like it or you don't like me, we'll figure out something else to do," This accomplishes several things. It takes the pressure off the first session and off the client, who now can afford to be less vigilant and wary of you. In the promise of such a short time limit is a protection against the loss of precious autonomy. It also gives you time to prove that you are someone who is easy to talk to, who really can understand the nuances and implications and dilemmas the client brings to you, and who is interested in improving your client's life.

Obviously, this promise of a time limit may not always be possible because of limitations under which you work. If the client has been mandated by a court to see you for a specific number of sessions, your hands may be tied. In most cases, however, you will not be the only mode of treatment available. So when you say, "We'll figure out something else to do," you might have in mind or even explicitly name what some of those alternatives might be. In essence, you are saying to your client, "I understand that you're here because you have to be and you have to get some kind of help, but it doesn't necessarily have to be me. Let's give it three sessions and see what happens. If it doesn't work out between you and me, you might join an anger management group at the clinic [or whatever alternative treatments are available]." There certainly is a complex and difficult issue around giving the client this kind of control, but my experience is that three sessions of good therapy can engage many involuntary clients, and if, after three sessions, an involuntary adolescent client still doesn't want to talk to me, it's unlikely that treatment will be successful anyway.

Termination Issues

One of the most gratifying and most difficult aspects of working with adolescents is ending a relationship, particularly a long one. The ideal termination is one in which you and your client mutually recognize that progress has been made toward relief of the problems that brought the client to therapy; your client feels stronger and in less need of therapy. Your client thinks of you as a trusted adult but is ready to move on with his or her life. You make a mutual decision that it is time to end treatment.

The reality of doing clinical work with adolescent clients is far messier that this. Many terminations result from adolescent clients simply quitting treatment, running away, or deciding not to cooperate. Sometimes parents become frustrated with a perceived lack of progress or are threatened by a strong relationship between the therapist and the client and force a termination of treatment. Sometimes funding for treatment runs out, and often a time-limited program comes to an end, such as at the end of the school year. The world of clinical work with adolescents is simply more tumultuous than the world of clinical work with adults. You need to be ready for considerable frustration over unsatisfactory terminations. Of course you need to be optimistic and positive about your work, but you also need to be realistic. Most of the people I know who work with adolescents do not think in terms of a cure or completed treatment when they do personal evaluations of the impact of their work. They think more in terms of, "Have I had some positive impact in changing the direction of this young person's life?"

Laying Groundwork for Termination from the Beginning   In many places throughout this book I discuss the importance of being clear about the limits of the treatment relationship. One of the most important reasons for being clear and straightforward about your role in the client's life is to prevent problems around termination. It is not that the clinician frequently and strongly makes a big issue of this, but it is always implicit and sometimes spoken about that the client and the clinician have a strong, warm, accepting, and empathic relationship but that the clinician is not and will not be part of the client's life outside treatment. You are your client's *clinician,* and that's a wonderful and important and powerful thing to be. But treatment does not last forever, and your job is to help your client build an effective life outside treatment. If you promise, implicitly or explicitly, to be more than you are, you will inevitably hurt some clients. In essence, you try to minimize feelings of abandonment at termination by being clear about your role in the client's life.

You also lay groundwork for termination by being open to talking about it whenever the issue comes up or whenever your client hints at thoughts related to termination, such as the future, your long-term place in the client's life, and abandonment.

Teaching and Giving Information

I have already discussed the risks and benefits of giving an individual client advice, and some of the same principles apply to the more formal situation in which we want to teach the client something.

When Teaching Is Appropriate   As with giving advice, the basic principle for deciding when direct teaching is appropriate is to ask yourself whether you have information that the client does not have or cannot figure out. Whenever possible, it is far more powerful and effective to help your client think through and solve his or her own problems. It is often difficult to watch a young person struggle with this problem-solving process, and it is terribly tempting just to tell him or her the "truth." If you do this when your client could have figured things out, you have taken away an opportunity to become stronger. Emotional problems impair problem solving, usually not because the person lacks information or cannot get the necessary information but because anxiety and other emotions interfere with thinking and experiencing accurately. One of the most important goals of therapy is to enable the client to do this accurate thinking and experiencing. On the other hand, in some situations it would be foolish and almost cruel to let a client struggle hopelessly in the absence of critical information. The trick, obviously, is deciding when your opinions and information are just providing something your client doesn't have access to.

I am making an issue out of this partly because almost all of us have a strong tendency to try to fix young people. We want to give advice, teach, and lecture. These things come easily to us, and they are among the most common social behaviors that life seems to teach us. Finding ways to facilitate a young person's own growth processes is far more difficult but far more helpful.

Having said all this, however, I can now present some specific programs that are largely based on teaching such things as behavioral principles, social skills, and anger management. Our job as clinicians is always to have in mind that whatever teaching we do, we do in the service of enabling the client's own problem solving.

BEHAVIORAL INTERVENTIONS

Behavior therapy (also called behavior modification) is both widely used and widely misunderstood in the treatment of adolescents. The principles of learning on which behavior therapy is based are both powerful and complex. These principles can be effectively applied in hundreds of different ways. Thus I do not focus on specific techniques here but instead focus on understanding the fundamental principles and seeing how they can lead to a wide variety of techniques. For specific techniques I recommend reading the books by, for example, Martin and Pear (1998) and Spiegler and Guevremont (1998); a well-trained clinician should learn some of the specific techniques.

In general, the techniques can be divided into three approaches: (1) desensitization methods designed to reduce undesirable emotional reactions, such as fear and anxiety, through extinction (exposure to the feared stimulus with no aversive consequences) and/or counterconditioning (exposure to the feared stimulus along with positive consequences and responses that are incompatible with fear); (2) operant or positive reinforcement methods, which use rewards to establish desirable behavior; and (3) aversive conditioning, which uses punishment to eliminate undesirable behaviors. The first two approaches are effective in the treatment of clearly definable behavioral problems. Aversive methods, however, are rarely used today and are effective only as a part of treatment that includes much positive reinforcement.

Within these three broad categories it is difficult to specify a short list of particular techniques. Rather, the emphasis is on principles of learning, and specific techniques are limited only by the imaginative application of the principles to the complexities of individual cases.

Basic Principles of Learning

It would take many books to explain all the principles of learning, but I briefly mention a few of those principles that you are likely to use in carrying out a treatment program with adolescents.

Principles of Reinforcement and Punishment   Probably the most useful principle in behavior theory is that people do what they are reinforced for doing. This principle may seem blatantly obvious to you, but few people understand all its implications. We often attribute the behavior of others to such things as laziness, foolishness, good heartedness, and hundreds of other personal motives and qualities. The learning theorist says that whatever a person is doing, he or she is somehow being reinforced for doing it. This insight provides a powerful principle for how to change behavior: Change the reinforcers.

In life, however, this simple-sounding principle is incredibly complex and difficult to apply. Many people have an oversimplified understanding of reinforcement principles and focus on such reinforcers as money, food, and praise. It is possible that for some individuals praise is a punisher and being scolded is reinforcing.

Positive reinforcement is roughly synonymous with rewards, and *negative reinforcement* results when we withdraw pain or discomfort. Notice that negative reinforcement is not the same as punishment; they are commonly confused. Both negative and positive reinforcement are called reinforcement because they strengthen whatever behaviors they follow. In a sense, both are rewards. This is more obvious with positive reinforcement, in which we provide a consequence to behavior that feels good. Negative reinforcement is also a reward in the sense that it feels good for something painful to stop.

One kind of negative reinforcement is especially important in understanding our clients' disturbed behavior. Reductions of fear and anxiety are powerful negative reinforcers that often establish and maintain problematic behavior. For example, when a friend of mine and I were interns, we treated a boy who repeatedly rubbed bleeding sores on his arms, reopening the wounds. While others were healing, he reopened old lacerations and had no idea why he did this. We were sure, however, that this punishing behavior was somehow being rewarded by a powerful reinforcer, most likely the avoidance of something that was horrible and anxiety arousing to the boy. We did not know what this was, but there were dozens of possibilities. He might have felt deep guilt that was relieved by punishing himself in this way. He might have unconsciously feared that his parents would break up, and his bleeding arms distracted him from this (and maybe even helped keep his parents together as they focused on his problems). Thinking in terms of reinforcement helps us at least see that behavior that seems unusual is at least understandable.

Punishment is designed to decrease behavior, and it obviously can do this under the right circumstances. It involves the delivery of aversive consequences following a particular behavior. For our purposes in designing treatment programs for adolescents, however, using aversive consequences as a central part of the treatment program presents two big problems. First, punitive approaches almost inevitably elicit angry resistance from adolescents and, second, punishment works, in general, by suppressing the punished behavior, not by weakening or eliminating it. The punished behavior seems to disappear, but in fact what has happened is that a new behavior has been learned—that of stopping the punished behavior. The punished behavior is not weakened in strength at all, and thus if the inhibiting behavior is somehow lessened, the punished behavior that seemed to disappear will reappear at the same strength as if it had never been punished.

It would be naive to think that the treatment of adolescents could be carried out with no use of some kind of punishment, and earlier in this chapter I discussed circumstances that require the clinician to deliver consequences to clients. The primary principle I discussed was the delivery of natural consequences, as opposed to arbitrary punishments.

An understanding of reinforcement and punishment leads us to understand that the most effective way to influence behavior in the long term is to provide much positive reinforcement for desired behaviors combined with mildly aversive consequences for undesired behaviors. Using punishment alone will not establish new behaviors, and using reinforcement alone is often inefficient.

Principles of Fear and Fear Reduction   Many, if not most, of the problems you will encounter in your clinical practice are based on fear, using a broad definition of fear that includes negative, painful emotions, such as anxiety, depression, guilt, and apprehension. Before I discuss these more complex problems, it would be helpful to review a few of the simple behavioral principles of fear. An understanding of these principles will help you understand your clients' experience better and will help you design potential treatments. These basic principles may seem oversimplified to the point of simplemindedness, but they can tell us a great deal about the foundations of complex human experiences.

Learning theory says that the baby is born fearing nothing that is not physically discomforting. Through conditioning experiences based on the pairing of physical discomfort (pain, usually) with objects or even with his or her own behaviors that were originally emotionally neutral, the baby develops fears of those objects or behaviors. Once the child learns the powerful lesson of imitation, fears can also be acquired vicariously from the fearful reactions of significant others. Although the process here is more complex than with simple fears, the principles are still the same. Fears are fundamentally learned from association with physical discomfort

These simple principles can account directly for only the most obviously acquired fears, however, and most of the fears and anxieties that you will encounter in your adolescent clients do not easily fit the model of directly conditioned fear based on painful experiences. If you have a client who is afraid of cats or elevators or automobiles, it is most likely that these fears developed in a more complicated way than through a simple traumatic experience with these objects. We will try to understand some of these complexities.

One implication of the observation that all fears are learned is that, in principle, they can all be unlearned. It is extremely important that we understand that the evidence on conditioned fears tells us that the only way to weaken a fear is (1) to face whatever arouses the fear, (2) to feel the fear, and (3) to have no painful consequences associated with the experience. This process is called *extinction*, and it has enormous implications for how we treat emotional problems. We sometimes think that we can simply talk a person out of an unreasonable fear, but the principle of extinction tells us that the treatment process must be both cognitive and experiential. Felt emotion must also be part of the process. I will return to the implications of this principle.

There are at least four factors that make fears last for a long time in humans. Time, they say, heals all wounds, but that is not true of painful conditioned responses. The only way to get rid of a fear is to face it, feel the fear, and have nothing bad happen. Unfortunately (or probably fortunately for survival of the species), fears simply extinguish more slowly than other conditioned responses. A second, related factor is that humans quite understandably avoid the things they fear, and this prevents extinction from taking place. In fact, avoidance behavior is often strongly established and under conscious control, whereas the emotional reactions themselves take a few seconds to get started. Thus we can avoid feared situations so quickly and efficiently that our fears never extinguish unless circumstances force us into contact with the sources of our fears. The third factor is that avoidance behavior becomes extremely strong because every time we avoid something we fear, we feel better. Fear reduction is a powerful reinforcer, and the avoidance behavior becomes difficult to change. Fourth, the experiences that cause fear are usually unpredictable. This kind of partial reinforcement results in reactions that are resistant to extinction. The unpredictability comes both from the inconsistency of the persons doing the punishing and because we occasionally fail to avoid the real source of the fear; the unconditioned source of pain is so punishing that the fear is strengthed by another experience of conditioning. These occasional failures to avoid are unpredictable and establish the fear and the avoidance behavior even more strongly.

Finally, to really understand fear and anxiety, we need to know that it is almost universal among humans that we learn to fear our own thoughts, memories, and feelings. I suspect that you have had the experience of being alone, thinking some particular thought or memory, and feeling awful or embarrassed or frightened. You must have been aroused by your own painful thought. Understanding this principle helps us to understand one way it can be helpful for an adolescent to talk openly and freely with someone who both understands and accepts him or her. In terms of behavioral principles, what happens is that during the talking, the client exposes him- or herself to frightening thoughts, memories, and feelings in a safe, accepting atmosphere. The client feels some discomfort from facing these feared internal processes, but extinction can take place and thoughts that used to be too painful to think lose their aversive power.

Applying the Principles

As I noted at the beginning of this section, the application of behavioral principles requires creativity on the clinician's part. There are hundreds of possible ways to apply the principles. Behavioral treatment, however, can be divided into three general areas: (1) desensitization methods; (2) contingency based methods, that is, the use of reinforcement; and (3) aversive methods, that is, the use of punishment.

Exposure Methods for Desensitization Desensitization techniques are designed to reduce aversive emotions, especially fear. Desensitization requires three components: (1) The person must face the feared object, situation, thought, or feeling; (2) the person must experience the fear, preferably in small steps; and (3) this experiencing should be accompanied by no bad consequences or, even better, positive consequences. The specific techniques designed for desensitization are usually referred to as *exposure methods*, because the critical element is the exposure to whatever causes the fear.

A critical phrase from the previous paragraph is "preferably in small steps." Some exposure programs use flooding techniques, in which a client is suddenly and intensely exposed to highly fear arousing stimuli. This may work in some circumstances, but it also carries considerable risk of causing new fear conditioning in which the original fear is intensified or new objects become sources of fear. Most exposure treatments are based on *graduated extinction*, in which the person is exposed to mildly fear arousing stimuli first. When the client becomes comfortable under these circumstances, he or she is exposed to the next step in a hierarchy of situations or objects that are arranged from less fear arousing to more fear arousing.

A practical example of graduated extinction is that of a young woman who was in a car accident and subsequently was too frightened to ride in cars. Once her therapist explained the principles of graduated extinction to her, she was able to plan and execute her own treatment program, in which she started out by simply getting into and out of a car. She understood that each step she took was to push her to her edge of anxiety, a place where she felt some fear but not so much that she couldn't complete the act. Eventually, getting into and out of a car became so easy it was almost boring, and she was able to ride in the passenger seat while an adult slowly drove the car around an empty parking lot. By doing each step until it became relatively free of fear, she was eventually able to resume riding in cars. The beauty of this example is that her therapist taught her the principle; she gave the girl a tool to use, and the client not only dealt with her fear but also had the empowering experience of, "I did this myself."

An important caution is to realize that most intense fears do not have as simple a causal history as a fear of riding in a car that results from being in an accident. For example, one adolescent boy was afraid to stay overnight anywhere other than his home. This fear prevented him from participating in many experiences that he wanted, such as going to camp. We could devise a graduated extinction program in which he might stay at the next-door neighbor's house one night and then gradually progress through more and more difficult situations. Such a program could well be a helpful part of treatment, but it is unlikely that the causes of his fear are this simple. His fear of staying away from home might involve other issues of which neither he nor we are aware. For example, he might have some deep fears of abandonment that become active without his awareness when he is away from his parents, or he could fear losing control of his emotions in a strange situation. The problem, obviously, is that it is often difficult to identify the real causes of intense fears. My preference is to combine talking therapy with providing my client with behavioral tools to use in creative ways.

Counterconditioning is also used in desensitization. The feared object or situation is presented simultaneously with an incompatible positive stimulus, such as deep relaxation, good food, or anything that induces a positive feeling. There is a subtle but important difference between counterconditioning and extinction. Extinction actually weakens fear. In its pure form counterconditioning competes with and suppresses the fear, but it does not actually weaken it.

In practical applications we are almost always using both extinction and counterconditioning because a client is exposed to the source of the fear, feels the fear, and has new positive feelings in a safe setting. The important lesson to learn is that for this process to work, the client must feel the fear. If you are afraid of flying and you take powerful tranquilizers that make you feel wonderful every time you fly, you will not get over your fear because you prevented yourself from feeling it. Even though the pleasant feeling from the tranquilizers is associated with flying, your fear is only temporarily suppressed, not weakened.

Contingency-Based Methods   Behavior therapists strongly emphasize the power of positive reinforcement. People do what they are reinforced for doing, and, in general, if you want to change behavior, you should change what reinforces the behavior. This relatively simple principle is enormously complicated in application, but two observations are of special interest to us as clinicians who work with adolescents.

The first observation is that many people have a simplistic idea of how reinforcement works. They think in terms of external or *extrinsic reinforcement*, such as giving money for good grades or candy for good behavior. It is far more powerful to plan *intrinsic reinforcement*, such as promoting social interaction by making the social interaction itself pleasurable. For example, we could offer a group of young clients movie passes if they avoid fighting with each other for three hours. On the other hand, we could plan an activity that is intrinsically fun only when they are not fighting. In the first case the effect of our reinforcers is likely to be temporary, because the reward for not fighting is extrinsic. When the extrinsic reward is no longer available, there's no reason not to fight. In the second case the effect is likely to be more long lasting.

The second observation is one I have mentioned before: One of the most powerful reinforcers in human experience is *anxiety reduction*. Many of the self-destructive things that adolescents do they do because these behaviors bring immediate reduction of loneliness, fear, a sense of not belonging, and many other painful emotions. This immediate reduction of painful emotions is so powerful that, even if a behavior leads to serious trouble down the road, it is still worth doing. The point is that it is not sufficient just to stop the self-destructive behavior. We need to think in terms of making alternative, prosocial behaviors powerfully and immediately reinforcing.

The Most Powerful Way to Influence Behavior   Because it is such an important principle, I am going to repeat a paragraph from a previous section. An understanding of reinforcement and punishment leads us to understand that the most effective way to influence behavior in the long term is to provide much positive reinforcement for desired behaviors combined with mildly aversive consequences for undesired behaviors. Using punishment alone will not establish new behaviors, and using reinforcement alone is often inefficient.

Our culture seems to act as though punishment were the most effective tool for change, but it only teaches what *not* to do, and it has many destructive side effects when it is the primary tool used to influence behavior. People, including adolescent people, mostly do what is rewarding to them.

COGNITIVE BEHAVIORAL THERAPY

Cognitive behavioral therapy (CBT) has become one of the most popular and widely researched approaches to treatment. It was originally designed to add a needed complexity to early versions of behavior therapy, which focused primarily on factors external to the client. Cognitive behavioral theorists argue that thinking is probably the most important human behavior. They say that thinking is best understood as a kind of behavior that may go on inside a person's skin but that it is still behavior and it still follows the same principles and laws as other more observable behaviors.

In essence, cognitive behavioral theory says that maladaptive behavior and painful emotions are largely the result of distorted cognitions. Following from this, CBT is aimed at understanding and correcting these distorted cognitions. One of the most powerful forms that these cognitions take is that we all develop schemas in our thinking patterns. These schemas are similar to generalized categories or templates that structure our thinking. For example, each person has a unique "new social situation" schema. We have a generalized picture of what to expect from ourselves and from other people in a new social situation. This generalized picture saves us a lot of time processing all the new information bombarding us in a new social situation, but it also means that we will inevitably distort our perception to some extent to fit our schema. One person's schema might be built around an expectation that new social situations are somewhat dangerous, whereas another person's schema might include the expectation of new friendships as central. These expectations strongly affect the perceptions and behaviors of a person, and to the extent that they are distorted, they can cause painful emotion and maladaptive behavior. CBT is often designed to change schemas.

Another helpful concept is that of core beliefs. We all have hundreds of schemas, but some of them are relatively minor and some are fundamental to our perception of the world. The cognitive behavioral therapist tries to understand and focus on the client's core beliefs, because correcting distortions in these schemas will have the greatest impact on improving a client's life.

In its most strongly stated form, cognitive behavioral theory argues that cognitions cause emotions. Ellis's (1994) rational-emotive theory, for example, flatly states that reason controls emotion and that faulty emotions are entirely the result of faulty reasons or beliefs. Other versions of cognitive behavioral theory, however, include some version of what sounds like unconscious causes of emotions, such as automatic thoughts and schemas of which the client is not fully aware.

Cognitive behavior therapists have developed a range of techniques and methods, and there is considerable evidence that these techniques are helpful, especially with depression but also with many other disorders. Lewinsohn and Clarke (1999) examined CBT for adolescent depression in 12 different studies and concluded that "63% of the patients showed clinically significant improvement at the end of treatment. Clearly, the treatments have a large effect" (p. 337).

It would be impossible to describe all the potential CBT methods because there are so many ways that the basic principles can be applied. I describe several creative ways that CBT has been used with adolescents, partly to provide you with some specific techniques but, more important, to give you examples of how the principles can be applied. You, of course, can creatively develop unique applications that fit your unique situation and clients.

Correcting Some Common Misconceptions

Before we get started with that, however, a few cautions are in order. Some people misperceive CBT to be a relatively simple process in which the therapist changes the client's thought patterns.

First of all, CBT is primarily a *collaborative process* in which the clinician and the client work together, primarily to facilitate the client's own problem solving. Obviously, this collaborative approach is consistent with the perspective of previous chapters, and it is important that CBT not be seen as something the clinician does to the client.

Second, CBT involves a complex process of talking, through which the therapist and client make discoveries about the client's beliefs. One cognitive behavior therapist I know says that he attunes himself with the client as part of the process of discovering the client's core beliefs. He provides his clients with a remarkably deep understanding. David Burns, one of the best known cognitive behavior therapists, has reported (Burns & Nolen-Hoeksema, 1991) that one of the most important aspects of CBT is therapeutic empathy, as measured by client reports of how deeply understood they felt: "The causal effects of therapeutic empathy on recovery appear to be large" (Burns & Auerbach, 1996, p. 161).

Third, some presentations of CBT seem to imply that changing cognitions is the whole story in treatment. However, there is considerable evidence that effective treatment combines both cognitive and experiential elements (Martin, 2000; Bohart, 1993). Another way to say this is that the process of treatment is both cognitive and emotional. This is strongly supported by the discussion of extinction principles in the previous section. In addition to the evidence on how extinction works, there is considerable evidence that reason and emotion are separate systems in humans. Reason clearly influences (and often distorts) emotion, but it is also true that emotion and experiential knowing clearly influence (and often distort) reason (Bohart, 1993; Toth & Reingold, 1996; Vanaerschot, 1997).

CBT Techniques

Cognitive behavioral therapy lends itself to relatively highly structured treatment programs that are combinations of direct teaching and therapeutic discussion. Many of the programs use detailed treatment manuals, and some of them have been developed specifically for adolescents (Hibbs & Jensen, 1996). One of the most creative applications of cognitive behavioral principles to the treatment of adolescents is the book *Tough Kids, Cool Counseling* (Sommers-Flanagan & Sommers-Flanagan, 1997).

Lewinsohn and Clarke (1999) categorized CBT techniques used with adolescents in research studies into four general categories: (1) cognitive techniques, (2) family context treatments, (3) behavioral techniques, and (4) affective education and management. I briefly describe examples of each category.

Cognitive Techniques   Cognitive techniques are most closely identified with CBT. In general, they are designed both to correct distortions in cognitions and to modify cognitions in a positive direction, with the goal of creating positive emotions.

As the cognitive behavior therapist becomes familiar with a client's core beliefs, he or she starts to identify distortions. A young client might consider herself unattractive or might think that no one can be trusted, and these beliefs could be leading to both negative emotion and maladaptive social behavior. In CBT the therapist might challenge these beliefs and might assign the client homework to test them. For example, the therapist might suggest that the client keep a record of how attractive she thinks the other females around her are and thus discover that her standards for attractiveness are unrealistically high. Or the therapist might suggest that the client make up three lists of people labeled "completely untrustworthy," "somewhat trustworthy," and "trustworthy," with the goal of discovering that the belief that no one can be trusted is an overgeneralization, a distorted cognition.

Methods to empower clients and to teach them self-control rather than dependency on the guidance of others are central in CBT.

One of the principles of CBT is that many stressful and threatening situations are made more stressful by our cognitive evaluations of them. The principle is that nothing is good or bad, but thinking makes it so. Clients are often taught how to cope with stressful situations by using cognitive reevaluation methods.

It is often helpful to clients to learn behavioral principles, such as those discussed in the previous section, and how to apply those principles to changing one's own life. For example, a client who wanted to change a particular behavior might be taught reinforcement principles and then develop a personal program in which reinforcement is more consistently given for a desired new behavior.

Family-Oriented Techniques   Cognitive behavior therapists incorporate a wide range of methods, and these frequently include family interventions, such as conflict resolution, communication skills training, and parenting skills training. Many of these techniques were not developed directly by cognitive behavior therapists, but CBT draws from any source whose techniques are effective and consistent with CBT principles.

Behavioral Techniques   CBT often integrates the general principles of learning with the more cognitively oriented principles of CBT to teach problem-solving skills, social skills, and self-improvement to clients. For example, the therapist might recommend increasing pleasant activities in the client's life as a way to change mood and emotion. Similarly, the therapist might help the client set up situations in which he or she can experience small but significant successes as a way to build confidence and empower the client. Sommers-Flanagan and Sommers-Flanagan (1997) often teach strategic skills to adolescents. In essence, they help their clients identify desired goals and then to identify ways that the client's own behavior prevents achievement of these goals. For example, acting-out behavior usually leads to a restriction of freedom for disruptive adolescents, even though freedom may be the thing they want most. The therapist first establishes with the client that the therapist wants to help find ways to achieve the goals the client desires (within clear limits that exclude illegal or self-destructive behaviors) and then helps the adolescent explore his or her own behavior in strategic terms. "The strategic skills intervention is designed to help adolescents understand how their own behavior contributes to their inability to attain personal goals (e.g., perhaps by producing increased limits and restrictions)" (Sommers-Flanagan & Sommers-Flanagan, 1997, p. 114).

Affective Education and Management   A large number of treatment programs for changing emotions have been developed. Most of these programs draw from both cognitive behavioral theory and the general principles of learning. They include relaxation training, anger management, and mood management skills (Sommers-Flanagan & Sommers-Flanagan, 1997).

YOU NEED A LARGE TOOL KIT

I close this chapter by reminding you that being a clinician who works with adolescents requires both personal skills and a complex understanding of potential techniques. More important, you need to understand the principles behind the techniques because you will have to invent your own collection of methods creatively and often on the fly.

Recommended Reading

Ammerman, R. T., & Hersen, M. (Eds.). (1997). *Handbook of prevention and treatment with children and adolescents.* New York: Wiley.

Hibbs, E. D., & Jensen, P. S. (1996). *Psychosocial treatments for child and adolescent disorders.* Washington, DC: American Psychological Association.

Kendall, P. C. (Ed.). (1991). *Child and adolescent therapy: Cognitive-behavioral procedures.* New York: Guilford Press.

Sommers-Flanagan, J., & Sommers-Flanagan, R. (1997). *Tough kids, cool counseling.* Alexandria, VA: American Counseling Association.

Tolan, P. H., & Cohler, B. J. (Eds.). (1993). *Handbook of clinical research and practice with adolescents.* New York: Wiley.

Wilde, J. (1996). *Treating anger, anxiety, and depression in children and adolescents: A cognitive-behavioral perspective.* Washington, DC: Accelerated Development.

GROUP THERAPY CHAPTER 5

Up until this chapter my focus has been on the individual client, but a great deal of clinical work with adolescents is done in groups. In fact, group therapy is often the treatment of choice for adolescent clients for many reasons. The importance of peer relationships, difficult issues around trust of adults, the opportunity for shared learning, and the possibility of having a place where one belongs but can also be autonomous are all powerful advantages of group therapy. Stein and Kymissis (1989) go so far as to say, "It would be unthinkable to have an adolescent program without a group treatment component" (p. 69). Azima and Richmond (1989) add, "There is little doubt that group psychotherapy is the treatment of choice for most adolescents who are in the process of separation from parents and who rely strongly on influential peers for identification and direction. The peer group is the natural developmental habitat in which the adolescent manifests his struggle for independence, a separate identity, and a transitional model for adulthood" (p. xiv).

GROUP WORK

The typical format for group work with adolescents seems to be that one therapist meets with six to ten clients for at least an hour and a half, once a week. As I show, however, adolescent groups can take many forms and can include whole day outings, trips to the gym, and shared projects in addition to what we might think of as more traditional group therapy. I have called this section "Group Work" because of this enormous variety, and only some of the formats I discuss resemble traditional therapy.

There are significant advantages to having two therapists working with a group, but this arrangement usually occurs in training settings or in agencies where the economics of having two therapists are not so restricting. Group therapy is sometimes thought of as a cheap substitute for individual therapy, but each format has benefits and limitations that the other does not, and the benefits of group therapy are especially salient with adolescent clients. A discussion of these advantages and disadvantages will make more sense if we first look at what Yalom (1995) has called the curative factors in group therapy. Although Yalom was discussing group therapy for adult clients when he described these curative factors, they also apply to adolescent group therapy, with some of the factors being especially important.

Curative Factors in Groups

Yalom (1995, p. 1) divided the curative factors into 11 primary categories: (1) instillation of hope, (2) universality, (3) imparting of information, (4) altruism, (5) corrective recapitulation of the primary family group, (6) development of socializing techniques, (7) imitative behavior, (8) interpersonal learning, (9) group cohesiveness, (10) catharsis, and (11) existential factors. Some of these factors are available in both group and individual therapy, but some of them require group membership to occur. I examine each category in the following paragraphs.

The instillation of hope can come solely from the therapist's confidence and acceptance, but only in a group can the client see others make progress and hear them tell of gains made with problems similar to the client's. Obviously, this is especially true when the clients are adolescents and the therapists are adults, with whom the young clients are less likely to identify.

Similarly, universality refers to the discovery that one is not unique in having threatening thoughts and debilitating problems, a discovery that is more likely to be made in a group. Another way to state this is that the group normalizes many of the thoughts, feelings, and actions that the adolescent often feels are uniquely horrible to him- or herself.

Imparting of information simply refers to teaching about coping techniques, the dynamics of emotional adjustment, and the like. It can be part of the teaching aspect of either individual or group therapy, although in a group other clients probably can add information not available to the therapist. Because there are so many ways that adults and adolescents live in different cultures, the other clients in the group are likely to have more credible and accurate information about the adolescent culture. In any case adolescents are likely to perceive this to be true.

Altruism is an experience that the group member can have through helping another client grapple with problems. In a good group the members learn to become therapeutic toward each other, often giving empathy, caring, and honesty in a much more powerful way than the therapist can. Clients often see such things as just part of the therapist's job but, when given by another client, they see them as based only on a desire to help.

Only a group offers the possibility of a reliving of the complex kinds of relationships that exist in families, and Yalom (1995) believes that this reliving of family issues is often an important part of group therapy.

Clients are often assigned to group therapy after an intake procedure if a lack of social skills is an important part of their problems. The group offers a chance to learn to talk to several other persons and to be in a more reciprocal relationship better than individual therapy usually does.

Imitative learning is extremely powerful and occurs in both group and individual therapy. In a group, though, the client has several persons to imitate and, probably more important, has the opportunity to see and learn from the therapist's interactions with other clients. It has been my experience that clients steadily become more empathic with each other as group therapy progresses. The first few sessions are usually filled with advice giving, because each member is sure that the others could solve their problems if they would just try some fairly simple solutions. Later, however, clients come to show an appreciation for and communicated understanding of the other clients. I would hope that they are learning to be therapeutic, partly by imitation.

Interpersonal learning and relating can take place more in a group than in individual therapy, the limits of which usually make it a one-way relationship.

Group cohesiveness refers to a remarkable experience that develops in a successful group—a feeling of belonging to a group that is really important and trusting. This feeling is qualitatively different from having a good relationship with a therapist. They are both powerful but in different ways. "Our group" often becomes an important part of the person's life. The adolescent's need to belong is one of the most powerful dynamics of this stage of life, and simply being an accepted member of a group is often healing. Many times, for example, a young client will be quiet during group sessions but will still be gaining significant benefit. Much of this occurs through observation of the interactions of other people, but much of it also occurs because of the experience of being part of a cohesive group.

Yalom (1995) uses catharsis to refer to the emotional relief that follows talking out painful material, a process that also happens in individual therapy.

Finally, existential factors are mentioned as "almost an afterthought" (Yalom, 1995, p. 88) and center on realizing and accepting personal responsibility. These issues often come up among adolescents, who are struggling with such questions as, "What is the meaning of life?"

Advantages and Disadvantages

With this long list of advantages available in group therapy, you might wonder why anyone would do individual therapy at all, but there are clear advantages to individual therapy. In fact, my personal preference in treating most adolescent clients is for them to have both individual counseling and a chance to participate in some kind of group work, usually with a different clinician. Or, if the adolescent is in a group with me, I commonly refer them to another clinician for individual therapy. Some therapeutic processes seem more likely to occur in individual therapy. Acceptance and understanding from six people are surely more powerful than acceptance and understanding from one person, but they are also less likely to occur.

One problem with groups is that trust is difficult to build in even one other person, so clients frequently hold back in group therapy material they would have talked about in individual therapy, often for good reasons. Some therapists do damage, primarily those who are open and honest in an attacking way (Mohr, 1995; Lambert, Bergin, & Collins, 1977; Yalom & Lieberman, 1971), and the group therapist often has to deal with similar interactions between group members. In individual therapy, if the client perceives the therapist as empathic, accepting, and honest, a successful outcome is much more likely (Gurman, 1977). But Gurman says that what little evidence exists for group therapy suggests that this finding is much weaker in this treatment format. He speculates that group members' perceptions of each other as empathic, accepting, and honest will, if we ever have the data, turn out to be more important.

THE CLINICIAN'S METHODS

In group therapy the therapist has a special role but still is only one of several people with whom the clients interact. The relationships are much more complex. For example, the clients can be together against other clients, or the therapist often is a member of the group in a more personally involving way than in individual therapy. In addition, a group process is occurring at all times, and the therapist's job is often to comment on and intervene in this process. The clients are still the primary problem solvers and the therapist (and group members) still needs to be empathic, accepting, and honest, but much more is involved. In this section I discuss some of what that "more" consists of.

The Alliance

When I was in graduate school, I wanted to do my dissertation on group therapy with adolescents. One of my advisers told me that I had chosen the two most difficult kinds of therapy and combined them, and doing research under these conditions would mean that I would be in graduate school for the rest of my life. I took his advice and studied adolescent identity instead, but he had made an important point. I think that the reason group therapy with adolescents is so complicated is primarily because so many relationships are involved. In previous chapters I emphasized that the relationship is central in treating an individual. The same is true of group therapy with adolescents, except that the clinician must be aware of many more complicated dynamics and permutations of relationships. Building a personal alliance with each group member is still extremely important, but the therapist also must be involved to some extent in the kind of relationships that develop between group members.

In addition to everything else I have discussed about the nature of a good alliance, group therapy uniquely brings in the power of cohesiveness. The need to belong is so powerful for adolescents that when a feeling of "This is my group" develops, it becomes one of the most powerful, if not the most powerful, healing factors in treatment. My point is to sensitize you to the importance of the therapeutic alliance in your group. No matter how clever or powerful your other group therapy techniques may seem, they will have little effect without a good group alliance.

The Adolescent's Need for Structure

In chapters 2 and 3 I noted that the unstructured approach to individual therapy is often confusing and threatening to adolescent clients. This is also true for the group setting. In fact, it is almost certainly more true in the group setting, because an unfocused, ambiguous starting of a group process is especially anxiety arousing for young people who not only do not know what they are supposed to do but also cannot predict what the other members of the group are going to do.

Strome and Loutsch (1996) recommend a "structured, educative form of adolescent psychotherapy." They say that "although more classical techniques involving neutrality may work well with adult inpatient groups, . . . passivity and ambiguity on the part of the leader, coupled with an unstructured situation, produced high levels of anxiety and nonproductiveness in adolescents" (p. 176). In this chapter I discuss a number of kinds of structure that seem to work well in group therapy, in addition to the educative form that Strome and Loutsch recommend. Many of their observations are useful in understanding that a structured group does not necessarily mean a rigid, strict teaching situation. Because Strome and Loutsch believe in the importance of group members perceiving themselves as the agents of change in group therapy, they instituted practices such as making members responsible for bringing a topic for discussion to each meeting. They used role modeling, direct education, facilitation of discussion, limit setting, interpretive-like statements that were offered as suggestions or as personal reactions in a way that would reduce resistance, and judicious self-disclosure in a discussion format. They also said, "As important as, or even more important than, facilitating group process was the use of empathy in relating to others. Group members not only shared their impression of what might be going on with the other group members, but they were also encouraged to share similar feelings of their own" (Strome & Loutsch, 1996, p. 180). The structure that Strome and Loutsch brought to group therapy was to give the group members the assignment of bringing a topic for discussion to the session. This gave the adolescent clients enough "something to do" that they were not confused by ambiguity; there was a defined task. Then the arena was set for the therapists to work with whatever topics were brought in as the vehicle for therapy.

Empathy

Throughout this book I have stressed the importance and power of the experience of being understood by another person. In group therapy your adolescent clients will have an opportunity both to be understood by others and to be more empathic themselves. They will learn this partly by imitation of a skillful group therapist, partly from direct interventions by the therapist, and partly from other members of the group. In the beginning sessions of most groups there is a great deal of advice giving and confrontation. Even though each member of the group is struggling with his or her own issues that seem painful and daunting to that individual, often there is a lack of understanding for other people's problems. One young person might find it unbearably frightening to attend classes, whereas another might be self-destructively impulsive. It is not uncommon for the first one to say, "Well, why don't you just count to 10 when you feel yourself getting out of control?" The other one might later give the advice, "But there isn't anything to be afraid of in the classroom. All you have to do is be sure you sit near a friend." Each person finds his or her own problems overwhelming but has real difficulty empathizing with another person's problems as overwhelming. One common outcome of group therapy with adolescents is a significant increase in empathy among group members, assuming that the leader has maintained an atmosphere that encourages understanding.

A Place Where People Know Me   One of the curative factors in group psychotherapy mentioned by Yalom is group cohesion. Being a member of a cohesive group and having a strong sense of belonging in that group are probably more important during adolescence than at any other time of life. This sense of belonging has two primary components: being accepted and being understood. Receiving acceptance without feeling understood gives a young person the experience of, "Yes, you like me, but you wouldn't if you really knew me." The more thoroughly known or understood the adolescent feels in the group, the more important that group will be to the adolescent and the stronger the experience of curative cohesiveness.

Making Two People Feel Understood at Once   I have emphasized the fundamental skill of being able to make a young person feel deeply understood. As the leader of a group, you need this ability more than ever, and you need the ability to make more than one person at a time feel understood, even when they disagree with each other.

You might say, "I think Susan and Helen are talking about the same thing in some ways, but it feels very different to each of them. Susan, it's almost like you have felt so hurt by boys that it makes you want to just be alone, and I think it bothers you that Helen doesn't understand that hurt part. But Helen, you're sort of saying that even if a boy hurts you or tries to hurt you, it's important to fight back. It's almost like for you the anger is more important than that hurt, but that's not Susan's experience." The test of whether this response is on the mark or not is that we want each client to have the experience of, "Yes, that's exactly what I meant and how I feel about it." Just as if we were seeing an individual client, we want both Susan and Helen to feel deeply understood. But even more is happening here. Even though Susan and Helen disagree with each other, both of them are experiencing a third person who not only understands her but also understands and articulates the other girl's implicit message and experiencing. This process teaches a lot about empathy through the clinician's modeling, through hearing the other client's implicit message made explicit, and through the clinician's implied message that this kind of understanding between people is valuable and good.

Empathy between Adolescents in a Group   There is another, more direct way to facilitate empathy between the members of a group. Done clumsily, this way of facilitating empathy can come across as confrontational and judgmental. Done well, it can teach young people one of the most valuable relationship skills they will ever learn. In essence, the group leader asks one member of the group what he or she thought another member was trying to say or how the other member felt. Obviously, doing this could easily be perceived as a challenge or a test of the first person's ability to understand. Thus it needs to be done with sensitivity and with an easy way out if the first client is struggling with the question.

Commenting on Group Process

In addition to responding to the content of what group members say, the group therapist can be helpful by commenting on how the members interact with each other. As with all interpretations, these comments are offered in the spirit of tentative observations and educated guesses. They are offered as something for group members to think about rather than as statements of fact.

Common Threads and Shared Experiences   The therapist might say something such as, "It seems to me that several of you are saying a similar thing in different ways. There is kind of a theme about how parents seem to promise things that they don't follow through on." This one statement can make several of the clients feel understood, articulate an issue that several people may have only implied, and build feelings of cohesion and universality in the group as members see similarities between themselves and other group members.

Patterns of Communication   It is sometimes helpful to make a comment such as, "I'm not sure this is true, but it seems to me that whenever we start talking about going back home, this group gets pretty noisy." This identifies a repeated pattern of communication in a way that does not single out individual group members. It puts an observation on the table for the group to deal with or not, depending on whether they find it helpful. The clinician has not interpreted the meaning of the pattern observed, although a comment such as this clearly implies that there is some meaning to it. A similar example that focuses more on individual interactions but still without singling out individual people might be, "I think that most of us must expect criticism from others because sometimes it seems to me that in here we react like we're trying to defend ourselves, even when people say things that are not meant as attacks."

Preventing Damage   In some ways a group therapist is like a referee of the process. The therapist has to walk a fine line between facilitating and encouraging self-expression on the one hand and preventing group members from doing real emotional damage to each other with destructive attacks on the other hand. An important principle that you must teach by direct statement and example is that attacking another person's character and name calling are usually destructive; confrontations are an important part of our relationships, but they should be confrontations of what the person did, of the behavior. Especially in the early stages of group therapy adolescent clients will call each other stupid idiots, assholes, and much, much worse.

The potential for destroying trust and the fragile alliance building in your group is sufficiently great that you probably need to intervene to head off destructive attacks between members. However, it is almost useless simply to prohibit name calling and attacks. The most helpful strategy is probably to offer a reworded version of the

attack along with an explanation of why this wording is less destructive. You might say something to the effect of, "For sure we're
going to disagree with each other in this group and even have some
arguments, but it's really important that we try to avoid name calling when we do that. John, it's real clear to me that you think Robert
made a huge mistake by fighting with the policeman, but I would
rather you say something like, 'Fighting with a cop is stupid because you're sure to lose' rather than calling him a stupid idiot.
Does that make sense?" This comment accomplishes several purposes. It starts to teach John and all the other group members
something useful about confronting others, it offers Robert some
immediate relief and protection, and it helps to give all the group
members some increased sense of the group as a safe place to be.

Confrontation

Meyer and Zegans (1975) asked adolescent clients in group therapy
about their perceptions of therapy, and they concluded that group
members value clinicians who "manage that charmed balance between supportive care and objective discernment, between a willingness to interact emotionally with a young person and a respect
for his need for separateness and autonomy" (p. 22). This is a wonderful description of an effective group therapist with adolescents.
This description could apply in many places in this book, but for our
purposes I want to focus on the importance of combining supportive care and objective discernment. Objective discernment sometimes means that we need to confront our clients—sometimes about
things they have done and sometimes about ways we disagree with
them. Done well, confrontation can help a client grow and can even
strengthen the therapeutic alliance. Done poorly, clumsy confrontations are probably the most common way that clinicians alienate
young clients and damage the treatment process.

Stick to Events and Behaviors   In the previous section I discussed
the lesson you can teach your group members about confronting
others' behavior rather than their character. Obviously, you had
better live by this principle yourself when you confront group members. Few clinicians would call an adolescent client a stupid idiot or
an asshole, but it is discouraging to observe how many clinicians
do not realize that they are doing a slightly more refined version of
the same thing when they tell young people, "You're lazy" or "You're
too immature." There probably are situations in which generalized

attacks on character can be useful, but most often young people respond to them with enormous resistance, sometimes overt and sometimes hidden (and therefore maybe even more dangerous). The problem is that the adolescent finds an attack like this too big to deal with and too much of a threat to his or her whole person. If you confront or criticize specific events and behaviors, your client may not be pleased with you, but at least there is the chance of making constructive changes; specific behaviors are a lot more changeable than large personal characteristics.

Empathic Confrontations   Any confrontation will arouse some resistance, but this resistance can be reduced if the confrontation is preceded by or embedded in words that communicate understanding. If a young client in group is screaming how much she hates her sister but has misty eyes at the same time, some clinicians would point out the discrepancy with a confrontational interpretation such as, "You're screaming that you hate your sister, but the tears in your eyes tell me that that's not really what you feel." This clinician might feel brilliantly clever, but I can almost guarantee that contact with the adolescent will be lost, and other group members will become more wary of expressing emotion. This confrontation only confronts; it does not both confront and understand. The clinician might better have said, "It seems like you're feeling a whole mess of things. I hear the hating, and I also think I hear other feelings like pain or being upset. It's really tough for there to be so much going on all at once." The first confrontation denies the reality of part of the client's experience. Almost all adolescents will take serious offense at the implicit "You're wrong" part of their experiencing. Actually, in this case the clever therapist was almost certainly wrong in that he or she confronted a discrepancy in a way that seemed to say humans should only experience one emotion at a time or at least should not experience contradictory emotions, which is obviously nonsense.

Interpretation

Group therapists often find interpretations useful, but most of the principles for interpretations in group therapy are similar to principles I have discussed in previous chapters, so I do not dwell on them here. Just remember that an effective interpreter is not much more than an educated guesser. Interpretations are offered with skillful tentativeness. And this humble tentativeness is not based on a false humility; in fact, your interpretations will be wrong as often as they are right. If you are open to the ever-changing understanding of your young clients, you will discover that you will never have a client who doesn't surprise you at some point.

It is useful to remember Strome and Loutsch's (1996) description of

> interpretive-like statements . . . offered as suggestions or as personal reactions to minimize the resistance of group members. For example, when a patient was silent, angry, or dominated the session, the leaders made comments leading to self-examination. Comments such as "Kate, you seem very quiet today" or "Justin, I noticed that you're talking very rapidly. Are you aware of that?" were very helpful to both the individual and the group as a whole. If the group member was unaware of why he or she was acting in such a manner, the group members were asked to offer suggestions as to what they thought might be going on. (p. 180)

Eliciting Group Wisdom without Encouraging Attack Interpretations   This last suggestion by Strome and Loutsch nicely describes one way that interpretations in group therapy differ from individual therapy. Our primary goal is to help group members become more empathic toward each other, but interpretations and suggestions from one group member to another can be extremely helpful. The group leader sometimes needs to reword such interpretations or possibly to do some direct teaching so that interpretations between members do not become personal attacks. In a sense, the leader subtly teaches the value of skillful tentativeness and educated guessing so that group members offer each other interpretations and suggestions in a way that does not arouse resistance.

Blending a Focus on the Individual and on the Group

One of the most common errors made by group therapists is to do serial individual therapy, in which the therapist engages one client at a time in a process that strongly resembles individual therapy. It is important to blend work on individual issues with the involvement of the whole group or at least some other members of the group. Of course, sometimes it is necessary and most helpful to focus on one individual who is working through a particular issue, and the therapist will provide deep understanding, educated guesses, and affirmations of the client. As this process occurs, there are several ways to involve other members of the group. It is possible to say things such as, "That sounds a little bit like what Brenda was going through, but I see some differences too." Brenda may or may not respond at this point, but this kind of inclusive comment can be inserted subtly and still have a significant impact. Or the therapist might directly involve another client, provided that changing the focus does not interrupt an important process for the original group member. For example, you might say, "Brenda, does that sound similar to what you are going through?"

Another potential danger of serial individual therapy is that one or a few group members will dominate the discussion. The clinician should be sensitive to some sense of shared airtime among the group members who wish to talk.

Silent Members

One of the most important outcomes of good therapy with adolescents is simply to get them talking, especially to a trusted adult. This is not a superficial change in behavior; more thoughtful talking almost always means wiser problem solving and better relationships. Good therapy accomplishes this by making talking feel good. To state it in behavioral terms, if an adolescent is punished for talking (with scolding, judgment, or lack of understanding), he or she will talk less. If an adolescent is reinforced for talking (largely by being understood and affirmed), he or she will talk more. This is not a brilliantly complex concept, but most adults seem puzzled that adolescents will not talk to them. In group therapy the clinician's most important job is probably to get the members to talk. Many other activities are important, of course: providing information, working on issues, and all the methods and techniques I have discussed in this chapter. But our methods are nearly useless if group members feel threatened and clam up.

In a group silent members present a dilemma to the clinician. We cannot force them to talk. Actually, we probably can force them to talk but only in the short term, and we certainly will lose them in the long term. Usually, it is helpful near the beginning of a group to explain that no one will be forced to talk, although you hope that eventually everyone will feel comfortable talking in the group because that is the best way to get the most good out of the group. A skillful therapist can make this promise not to force talking with the confident knowledge that as he or she makes some individuals more and more comfortable talking, quieter members are also gradually learning that it is safe to talk.

Encouragement without Forcing   Keeping in mind that the first goal is just to get people talking, it is often helpful with quiet group members to encourage them to talk about something that carries little or no threat in the content. This can be as indirect as asking for concrete information, such as "Is it still raining outside?" More directly, a therapist can occasionally turn to a quiet member and say something to the effect of, "Nobody has to say anything they don't want say in this group, Chuck, but did you want to add anything to this?" The image I have in my mind as I write this is that Chuck probably will shake his head no and say nothing, and the therapist will gently move on to something else. But I hope that the therapist has gently invited him to join in without forcing. If and when Chuck does say something, the therapist will try to respond in a way that will make Chuck feel, "OK, he got that, and he didn't make a big deal out of it." It would be tempting to seize on Chuck's contribution and try to get him to say more, but that would be a little like hugging a kitten to death.

They Are Often Learning a Lot   One comforting observation is that silent group members are often listening hard and doing a lot of internal processing as they learn from the discussion of the group as a whole. My experience has been that as quiet group members become more verbal, they frequently make reference to material from previous sessions and to things they have learned from the group.

TYPES OF GROUPS

Many kinds of groups have been devised for the treatment of adolescents, partly to provide the kind of structure that adolescent clients seem to need, partly to adapt to different needs of adolescents at different stages of development, and partly to provide vehicles for treatment that are both verbal and nonverbal.

Activity Groups

Probably the most obvious example of providing a vehicle for treatment is the development of activity groups for adolescent clients. You often have to be *doing* something to engage an adolescent, and then you can form a relationship and work on issues.

Expressive/Creative Groups   Expressive groups use creative media such as film, drama, poetry writing, and art. These activities provide not only something to be doing together but also a nonverbal or symbolic language for expression. In a drama group, for example, it is possible to plan and act out a brief story that is not really about a specific client or his or her experience but through which feelings can be expressed indirectly. Sometimes, a drama group can act out for one of the members an incident that is really about that client's experience in a way that helps the person work through specific issues, rehearse different ways to handle a situation, or do some self-disclosing that is less threatening because it is "just pretend."

Obviously, writing poetry or drawing pictures in expressive groups is done in an atmosphere with as little judgment as possible. The point is not to produce good art or good poetry; the point is to say whatever you want to say.

Expressive groups often make good use of videotape machines. They might create and act out a story to be videotaped and then combine this effort with a visit to observe a professional television station in action.

Task Groups   Task groups are often misunderstood by outside observers as not really therapy, because they look so unlike the stereotype of treatment. Task groups are organized around a specific activity and can take any form, as long as they have an organizing purpose and provide an opportunity to form a relationship with the clinician, provide mutual listening, develop social and problem-solving skills, and relate to other adolescents. Examples of task groups are cooking groups, fitness groups, environmental groups, or store groups. In a store group adolescent clients are assigned the task, say, of organizing and operating a snack shop in their treatment facility. This process involves organization, problem solving, and enormous interpersonal learning in addition to the more obvious life skills of making financial decisions and running a business.

Some of the most powerful therapeutic moments you will have with an adolescent client, both in group therapy and in individual therapy, will happen in a seemingly offhand way as you are both engaged in an activity. Maybe your group will be making pizzas together, and one member will say, "This is the way my mom and I used to do it." You might gently ask, "Do you miss that?" "Yeah." An imported therapeutic moment has happened, and it has had an impact on most of the group members, who now have shared an important moment with the client who spoke. This is a subtle but powerful process.

Personal Exploration Groups

Personal exploration group therapy is sometimes also called inter-active group therapy. This is the kind of group that most people think of when they imagine group therapy. It usually consists primarily of regular meetings in which people talk about and explore situa-tions, feelings, and relationships. With adult clients such groups tend to meet over extended periods of time, and membership of the group may change as members leave and new people join. As I have said many times, however, adolescent clients tend to need more structure and predictability than adult clients, and so personal ex-ploration groups for adolescents are more likely to have a time structure that may be related to the school year, for example, and are usually presented in a less open-ended form.

A personal exploration group for adolescents is usually intro-duced to the clients with considerable explanation of the purpose and potential benefits of talking through issues rather than being started in an ambiguous way in which the clients structure the process. Although many adolescents have trouble getting involved in such a group, a significant number find the experience helpful. These clients tend to be somewhat older adolescents, are probably more verbally oriented than average, and have some psychological mindedness about their lives.

One of the most interesting and powerful aspects of personal exploration groups is that the process of mutual exploration, hon-est feedback from peers, and the formation of relationships within the group often become more important and more healing than dealing with any specific issue.

Psychoeducational Groups

Psychoeducational groups are designed to deliver specific informa-tion in a context that allows discussion of the importance of an ap-plication of that information to the clients' lives. Because group meetings involve a didactic component, the sessions are relatively highly structured. Normally, the didactic component is presented in the first part of the meeting through lectures, films, and written in-formation. Then there is a group discussion in which the leader fa-cilitates group members' reaction to the information, their relation of the information to their own lives, and the sharing of stories and experiences among themselves. Usually, group members have a shared concern and interest about the topic covered, and one of the most important outcomes of psychoeducational groups is the support that group members give each other. In many ways the group discussion is the more important part of these meetings.

Psychoeducational groups are almost always structured around a specific topic, such as assertiveness training for girls, avoiding unhealthy eating habits, anger management, moving to your own apartment, or transitioning from the hospital to a community school. Obviously, hundreds of other topics would also be appropriate for a psychoeducational group.

Theme-Oriented Groups

As with psychoeducational groups, theme-oriented therapy groups gather clients with a shared concern, life crisis, or personal problem. These groups, however, are less structured around teaching and imparting information and are more similar to personal exploration groups in that the focus is on mutual sharing of stories, mutual support, and problem solving.

Community Service Groups

One of the most powerful forms of an activity group for adolescents is the community service group. On the surface these groups look like simple work experience groups, but they provide the opportunity for many kinds of emotional and social healing for adolescent clients. In order for these groups to be more than simply work, they need to be designed around a guiding philosophy.

In the following section, Mitch Bourbonniere describes an especially successful community service group. He starts with an understanding of the most fundamental needs that young people bring to treatment and then shows how this understanding guides the design and functioning of the group. What Bourbonniere leaves out of his description (out of modesty, I suspect) is the importance of having an adult leader who both lives by a philosophy of community service and has the gift of connecting with adolescent clients at a deep level. Bourbonniere shows how community service groups meet some of the most basic special psychological needs of adolescent clients, which I discussed in Chapter 1.

COMMUNITY SERVICE GROUPS AND THE SENSE OF BELONGING, EMPOWERMENT, IDENTITY, AND PURPOSE

BY MITCH BOURBONNIERE

I believe that young people—adults too, for that matter—need to feel that they belong, that they have a sense of control and empowerment, that they have some measure of identity and independence, and that they have purpose and meaning.

A sense of these qualities can be instilled in people developmentally through a healthy family and a community environment. These qualities can translate into strength of character, resiliency, altruism, and, ultimately, positive self-esteem.

Unfortunately, some young people are exposed to less healthy environments and never get a chance to develop a strong sense of belonging, empowerment, identity, and purpose. Not only that, but many of them are left not feeling much of anything (other than a sense of having been ripped off). Whereas some children feel the safety and security and ultimately happiness of being part of their world, other children feel outside, alienated, unloved, unlovable. Some have no respect for a world that has not respected them. Rather than feeling good about themselves and ultimately going beyond themselves to empathize with and even serve others, they get stuck at much earlier stages, their emotional selves still crying out for what they did not receive, not seeing beyond themselves, and often wallowing in self-pity and selfishness.

The need for belonging, empowerment, identity, and purpose is like emotional food. People attempt to secure these by any means they can. Often people who have been deprived of a sense of healthy family and community will find one another. They don't feel worthy, deserving of, or particularly welcome to be part of more traditional groupings and instead form their own "families." These include gangs, street life, prostitution, the bar scene, drug culture, cults, Satanism, and other such groups. These groups are powerful and tend to lure vulnerable people with the illusion of belonging, power, identity, and purpose. As we all know, this illusion soon turns to more disillusionment.

Still, people are loath to leave these lifestyles because, as destructive as they may be, that is all they have. It is an anomaly; in order to survive, they engage in self-destructive behavior.

With these ersatz families being as powerful as they are and still offering a pseudo-sense of belonging, it is next to impossible to draw these people away from such lifestyles without offering an alternative. As a helper, I'm not powerful enough to prevent young people from doing drugs and alcohol, attempting suicide, or running in gangs. I can't be with my clients 24 hours a day. If they are intent on the behavior, no one can stop them. Even if I could stop them, what would that leave them with? In some ways, as dysfunctional as it is, they are simply trying to cope and survive. Maybe these self-destructive behaviors are what is allowing them to survive. Unfortunately, eventually it can also cause their demise.

Instead of stripping my clients of what they are using to survive and cope, I concentrate on offering them an alternative vehicle to feel a sense of belonging, empowerment, identity, and purpose. I form my own gang. I attempt to be just as hardworking and creative as the adults who "befriend" our vulnerable children, recruiting them with the promise of what society has failed them on.

The idea of a community service group evolved slowly into what is now a fully operational work experience program. Through word of mouth in the community, people call our group of young men to pick up donations of clothing, furniture, and household goods. These are then delivered to those in need, such as young people going into independent living, families relocating to the city, inner city families (including members of the group and their families), as well as refugee and immigrant families. Extras go to agencies and programs such as Habitat for Humanity and the Salvation Army and to many smaller local charities and programs. A relationship has formed between these families and agencies and our young men.

Other tasks the young men had been involved in include community cleanups, delivering fliers for charities, and mowing lawns and shoveling walks for the elderly.

Yet another endeavor includes the establishment of a recycling company. The young men negotiate and commit to servicing local businesses.

These young men seem to be benefiting on several levels. First, they are practicing having a job. They must show up for group or phone in. They learn about responsibility, accountability, and commitment. Once in attendance, they must work hard.

Second, they learn actual work skills—how to negotiate a business agreement, how to respond to a customer, how to maneuver a couch around a corner and up the stairs. In fact, sometimes when the work is particularly difficult, such as digging a trench, the members seem to realize that this is not what they might choose to do for a living. This invariably leads to a discussion on education and staying in school.

Third, they learn higher-level interpersonal skills. There are plenty of opportunities for these young men to practice anger and stress management, assertiveness, communication, problem solving, conflict resolution, teamwork, and team building and cooperation. In fact, socialization

continued

COMMUNITY SERVICE GROUPS AND THE SENSE OF BELONGING, EMPOWERMENT, IDENTITY, AND PURPOSE *(continued)*

is enhanced by the group members themselves. What has evolved is that more senior members pass on to newer members the norms and values of the group. Members don't want to be embarrassed in the community, and they certainly police one another.

The other way to enlist cooperation from the members is to give each member a sense of individual responsibility. One becomes the copilot in charge of map and directions; another ensures that we have the proper tools; yet another will be the front man in dealing with the customer. It always seems to work that the more potentially disruptive a member may be, the more responsibility you give him.

Fourth, they learn about the environment, about giving and receiving, about things coming full circle. They learn that for the most part, what you give out, you get back. This reciprocity is emphasized by the community families we serve insisting on feeding our young men. When we purchased work coveralls, some of the women at the family center we deal with offered to hem and make alterations. When a broken piece of furniture is rescued from the junk pile, a handyman at another family center offers to repair it (this salvaging aspect is not lost on these kids who see it as symbolic of their own lives).

This notion of reciprocity is also important in getting the neighbors of the treatment center to warm to the clients. There was a time when if anything happened in the neighborhood, our kids were blamed. Through community cleanups, open houses, barbecues, etc., this is changing. An example of making the first move includes the members of our group showing up at one of our neighbors' to repair large patio screens that had recently been slashed. Although we were not responsible for the damage, we made ourselves responsible for the repair. Some of our guys acknowledged that this type of act makes up for other damage they may have done in the past.

Fifth, and probably most important, the need for belonging, empowerment, identity, and purpose seems to be met. The members end up feeling that they belong to the group and to one another. They feel empowered with all the new skills they are learning. They seem to feel an identity within the group and as a group. In terms of purpose, they want to be productive. They don't want to be bored. I can't take my 6-year-old daughter to the grocery store without her insisting on pushing and stocking the cart. I think it is natural for young people to want to be part of the action. Lots of the kids who aren't in the group say to us, "Hey, how come I can't go with you guys to work?" The other part of purpose is going beyond yourself and concentrating on others. This too, I think, is natural. Our young people don't always want to be sitting around talking about themselves and their problems. They want to get out and do for others. The rush they get from giving to appreciative people is apparent. When we deliver toys and clothes to a refugee family and their children hug and cling to the legs of our guys, you can just see the light inside of them go on through their eyes. In fact, many of the young people I've talked to who do robberies and home invasions are not doing it for the money but for the rush. They want to feel something—anything. Sometimes that rush happens in our group.

A couple of nice by-products have evolved from our work. One is that we always reward the members' hard work with a good meal. We have become regulars at a couple of mom-and-pop out-of-the-way diners. When we walk in, it's a little like the television show *Cheers*, where everybody knows your name. One kindly proprietor even throws in a round of Twinkies "for the guys" for dessert. When the restaurant becomes busy, the members have been known to start pouring coffee and clearing tables. The theme of belonging and giving back seems to emerge everywhere we go.

The other development that has occurred is that others want to be charitable through us. Last year, a doctor at our treatment center funded and helped deliver a hamper to one of our families. This year, a group of nuns wants to fast one day a week and donate their meal money to our group so that we can purchase a hamper at Christmas for one of our families. Finally, one story stands out in that it emphasizes that everyone involved, the group and the community, benefits. An older gentleman in the treatment center's neighborhood had passed away. His adult children came from out of town to put his estate in order. We offered to help them, and they gladly accepted. We spent a few days together boxing and organizing the contents of the home. Memories of the man were shared. At the end of the process the family donated much of the usable goods to our group and ultimately to the community. We soon received a letter from the eldest son stating how healing it was for the family to have spent this time with our group.

It is often said, "You cannot love another until you love yourself." Maybe it's more like, "You cannot love yourself until you love another."

STAGES OF GROUP DEVELOPMENT

Adolescent groups face different issues at different times in their development. In the beginning members may be focused on getting to know each other and on learning to trust, but near the end issues of separation and potential loss will be more important. Several writers have tried to describe the stages that groups go through in group therapy, but most of these models have been applied to adult group therapy. Shambaugh's (1996) review of the literature on the development of adolescent groups gives us some useful guidelines of what kinds of issues to expect at different points in a group's life.

These stages are only general guidelines to major issues. In fact, groups sometimes return to an earlier stage, especially in response to changes in group structure and task, such as the introduction of a new member.

Shambaugh's Developmental Model

Shambaugh (1996) identifies four stages of groups: (1) negative orientation, (2) the working phase, (3) differentiation, and (4) separation. I explore each of these.

When young people join a therapy group, they frequently respond with resistance and mistrust of the new situation. Some models of group therapy call this the phase of resistance. Shambaugh calls it negative orientation. From the adolescent's point of view this makes perfect sense because the new situation feels potentially dangerous, and, as with all attempts by adults at treatment, it is a potential threat to the client's autonomy and independence. It is difficult enough for an adolescent to trust one or two other peers, to say nothing of the adult leader or leaders.

The group therapist has several sensitive tasks to perform in this stage, primarily around building rapport and a sense of trust. The clinician provides structure for the group by explaining the purpose and procedures of the group, by openly and honestly answering members' questions about the purpose of the group, and by setting and explaining the limits within which the group can operate. Because building a group alliance and a sense of cohesion and trust is so important in the beginning stages, the clinician should be especially focused on making each member of the group feel deeply understood and accepted. Ideally, the group members would also make each other feel understood and accepted, but this is seldom the case. With each member trying to establish a safe place in the group, group members can sometimes be hard on each other. As I mentioned in the section on empathy between group members, one common form of this is for group members to be dismissive of the seriousness of other members' problems. An example might be of a young person with a drinking problem saying to another member, "If your parents are so hard on you, why don't you just leave?" and then being offended and hurt when someone responds, "Well, alcohol is ruining your life, I don't see why you don't just stop drinking."

The clinician could accomplish several things with a response that makes both members feel understood and that gently points out the issue of how our own problems seem so different and more serious than the problems of others. An effective response might be, "I think that both of you feel offended that the other person doesn't really understand what it's like to be you. It's like she really doesn't understand how hard it would be for you to leave home, and [turning to the other member] he really doesn't understand how hard it is for you to stop drinking. Sometimes it's very difficult to know what it feels like to be another person." The clinician has accomplished several things here. Both group members probably felt understood by the clinician, both for how difficult their problems feel and for their immediate sense of feeling offended. Much of the judgment is taken out of what the clinician has said by the last sentence that expresses an understanding of why the members made the comments they did. In addition to all this, the clinician is modeling the kind of behavior that we hope will grow between the group members. In essence, the therapist does whatever encourages a building of trust and gradual involvement in the group.

Shambaugh (1996) argues that the second general stage of group development generally goes one of two very different ways: power and control or intimacy and support. Some groups focus on issues of status and rebellion, and the therapist typically takes a problem-solving stance in which the focus is on the immediate task of resolving power issues in the group while still allowing appropriate autonomy for the members. Other groups "proceed directly to the stage of intimacy, in which the group is a supportive place where personal issues are discussed" (Shambaugh, 1996, p. 71). Most clinicians find this second kind of group more rewarding to work with, because the atmosphere is less contentious and there's more opportunity to discuss and resolve personal issues from life outside the group. Shambaugh describes this kind of group as "an idealized family, with the therapist as a good parent" (p. 71).

The process of problem solving as a group gradually evolves into more and more individualistic functioning in which the members relate to each other and to the therapist as distinct individuals.

This is the differentiation phase. As each person gains more self-understanding, the therapist starts to function more as a resource person than as a supportive parent. Members of the group know each other well and are freer to explore individual issues that will range over a wide variety of topics of interest to adolescents.

The final psychological task of a successful group is often a painful one. As the group ends, the inevitable separation creates a sense of loss that often arouses resistance in group members. Because this sense of loss is so difficult, group members and even therapists sometimes have difficulty dealing with it openly. However, it is a necessary part of the termination of a group, and members often gain a lot as they review their group experience and sometimes reminisce about and relive group memories.

THE THERAPIST'S OWN ISSUES

A clinician's personal issues are always involved in clinical practice to some extent, but this may be most true in group therapy. In individual treatment it is easier to maintain a kind of blank slate status or to keep an as-if stance as the clinician explores the client's issues. Group therapy, however, demands a much more complex interpersonal involvement from the clinician. The dynamics of many relationships are swirling around you as you work in a group, and even when you are working with just one individual, you are having an impact on every other group member, each of whom is observing you and reacting to you as a person.

Blind Spots

We all bring our own personal needs, our relationship histories, and our distortions to our clinical work. Some of us have difficulty dealing with, or even perceiving, anger. Almost all of us struggled with relationships during adolescence, and it would be amazing if we escaped those struggles without any residual blind spots. Group therapy has a special power to revive old issues for clinicians, and it is important to be as aware as possible of how these issues affect you during treatment. Probably the most effective way to have this awareness is to seek out consultation or supervision, depending on what is available in your work setting. Sometimes a supervisor or colleague might observe your group in action and be able to serve as a helpful listener to you. If you can afford the luxury of a co-therapist, that person is often in the best position to be such a helpful listener.

Co-Therapists' Relationship

Having two co-therapists facilitate a group has both advantages and disadvantages. One of the most comforting advantages is that you have someone with whom to discuss your reactions to the group and who can help you explore your own blind spots. The process of group therapy is so complicated and there are so many interpersonal dynamics to track that it is often helpful to have two perspectives on what is going on in the group. For some groups, such as a men's group or a women's group, it is most appropriate to have two male or two female co-therapists. In a mixed-sex group, especially one based on personal exploration, there are real advantages to having both a female and a male co-therapist. Often, a client is more likely to feel that he or she has a friend in court more easily with a therapist of the same sex. In other cases it will be important for a young client to work things through with the therapist of the opposite sex. To the extent that group therapy is a corrective recapitulation of the primary family experience, having both a male and a female co-therapist can be especially important

You should also give some thought to the nature of the personal relationship between the two therapists. It almost always works better if both clinicians have compatible styles in therapy so that they are not at odds and trying to accomplish contradictory goals. If one therapist is considerably more confrontational or more supportive in orientation than the other, for example, the clients will inevitably pick up the tension in the relationship and react to it. If you and a co-therapist are conducting a group under supervision, the two of you will have an opportunity to discuss the dynamics of your own relationship with your supervisor. Even if you have no supervisor, you should set aside some time to talk not only about the dynamics of the group but also about the quality of your working relationship.

Co-therapy can be a powerfully creative and shared activity that builds a strong sense of connection and even intimacy between co-therapists. It is important to discuss and understand the personal implications of this. One of the curative factors for a young person in a group can be the reliving of family experiences. Especially when the co-therapists are a male-female team, the sense of family can be strong. It is not uncommon for adolescent clients to jokingly call one or both of the therapists Mom or Dad. Received with good humor and within appropriate boundaries this joking around can be positive and therapeutic. It also can strengthen the bond between the co-therapists. The important principle is to remember that this bond and intensity and sense of family are all good but always have an as-if quality to them. You are at all times a clinician to your clients and a professional colleague with your co-therapist.

ARE GROUPS YOUR NATURAL HABITAT?

To finish this chapter, you might think through your own strengths and weaknesses in terms of whether you would be most comfortable and effective working with groups or with individuals. Of course, most clinicians have opportunities to do both, but different people seem better suited to one or the other. I have heard it said that you must first learn individual therapy skills and then apply them in the group setting because group therapy is so much more complex than individual therapy. Of the clinicians I know, however, many of those who are most effective in groups have done relatively little individual counseling. Some of them especially enjoy the complicated action of a group but are uncomfortable one on one.

Recommended Reading

Azima, F. J., & Richmond, L. H. (Eds.). (1989). *Adolescent group psychotherapy.* American Group Psychotherapy Association Monograph 4. Madison, WI: International Universities Press.

Kymissis, P., & Halperin, D. A. (Eds.). (1996). *Group therapy with children and adolescents.* Washington, DC: American Psychiatric Press.

FAMILY THERAPY WITH ADOLESCENTS

CHAPTER **6**

One dissatisfaction that is often voiced with individual therapy is that it is removed from the client's life, especially when the client is involved in significant relationships. The argument is that the client cannot really change except in relation to those significant others, and this argument applies especially to adolescent clients who are still living with or at least deeply involved with their parents and siblings. Many of the adolescent clients you will see will have tumultuous family situations that may or may not be appropriate for family therapy approaches, in which you see entire families or some members of a family together. My focus in this book is on treating adolescent clients, not specifically on treating families. However, many times your work with an individual adolescent will be complicated by his or her family relationships. Sometimes parents and other family members will be enormously helpful and cooperative, but sometimes you will be painfully frustrated by making significant progress with a client who then returns to a destructive environment that seems to undo any good the treatment might have done.

Family therapy is primarily based on communication, and its effectiveness comes primarily from changing destructive patterns of communication between the members of the family. As we saw with group therapy in the previous chapter, the therapist's job is often to comment on the nature of the process and to change it directly. Thus a family therapist directs the treatment process more than an individual therapist does. The overall goal is for members of the family to become each other's therapists, in the sense that they are understanding and accepting of each other. You can think of the therapist as the hub of a wheel with a different family member at the end of each spoke of the wheel. At first, the communication flows from each individual through the therapist, who is listening to everybody. Later in therapy, the goal is for the communication to occur between the clients, with the therapist gradually fading out and becoming unnecessary. The clients will start listening to each other and risking communication with each other only as it becomes safe and rewarding to do so. You teach by your example of listening and by keeping the process going in positive ways.

In chapter 5, on group therapy, I told you that one of my mentors said that doing group therapy with adolescents combined the two most difficult kinds of therapy. This may be my personal bias, but I need to warn you that I think doing family therapy with families of adolescents is even more difficult. As with group therapy, family therapy involves several relationships with all of their permutations, and the therapist has to make several people feel understood and accepted at the same time as well as track and think about multiple issues. With families, however, you also have to cope with patterns of communicating that have developed over many years, intense emotions (almost always including hostility) that have a long history, and personal goals that are often in direct conflict with each other. Family therapy can be enormously rewarding, but it is not simple.

CO-THERAPY

In chapter 5 I recommended the use of male-female therapist teams for mixed-sex groups so that each client has a friend in court to facilitate the feeling of being understood. This is often an advantage of co-therapy. Another advantage is that, especially with families, the interpersonal dynamics are so complex and so often involve the therapist that it is easy to lose perspective on the process and feel overwhelmed. Having a co-therapist often permits one therapist to hang back, less involved, so that he or she can bring a different perspective to the process. In addition, it is often a rewarding shared experience for the co-therapists to be working together. Particularly with families, having a co-therapist helps, whether the therapists are of different sexes or not. The biggest problem seems to be economics. In private practice few families can afford two therapists at once, and the caseloads of many agencies are so large that co-therapy is not practical. This is an unfortunate reality, and so if you have a chance to do co-therapy, grab it.

THE FAMILY AS A SYSTEM

The fundamental principle that guides and justifies family therapy is that the people who live together are an interacting system, and changes in one part of a system cannot occur without changes in another part. Bell (1963) tells of his having to switch from the perspective that the client was a problem to the insight that "the family is the problem!" (p. 3). Systems theory argues that the whole is greater than the sum of its parts, and the family system contains unique elements that go beyond what each member brings to treatment.

One of the most interesting observations that illustrates the importance of seeing a family as a system was reported many years ago. Long before systems theory became central to the practice of family therapy, Burgum (1942) presented an article with the interesting title "The Father Gets Worse: A Child Guidance Problem." Burgum wrote about "several cases which showed a shift in intrafamilial relationships following the same general pattern: the father gets worse as the mother gets better" (p. 474). Burgum described this pattern in a way that clearly illustrates how we cannot treat one person in a system without affecting others in the system:

> The presenting problem is usually profound antagonism between mother and child. The father, usually a dependent, immature man, at time of referral, is the child's protector or lurks in the background; while the mother is usually an aggressive, dominating woman, who rejects the child. While she responds to treatment, the father begins to behave brutally and punitively. The improved relationship between mother and child threatens the father, it activates his own latent aggression against the child which hitherto found a vicarious expression through the mother, it stimulates his feeling of sibling rivalry in relation to the child through being displaced by him as favored sibling. The father's loss of status in being deprived of the role of the good parent is another important factor in his subsequent disturbance. (p. 474)

An Identified Patient or the Family as the Client?

Bell's realization that he had to switch his perspective from seeing the client as the problem to seeing the family as the problem illustrates an important principle that you will run into in many places. Family therapists often use the phrase "identified patient" to imply to everyone involved that, although one person has been identified as the focus of treatment, everyone in the system is involved in both the causes and the potential solutions to the problems. Usually, the reasons that the family is in treatment do center on the problems of their adolescent child, and thus one task of the therapist is to take the perspective—and help the clients take the perspective— that no one is the patient. The relationship is the focus of treatment. Often one or both parents or even the siblings will say that they are willing to come in if it will help the troubled adolescent. Sometimes therapists let such statements pass, as a means of engaging the reluctant family member, but the perspective should be shifted to the family relationship as soon as possible without driving anyone from therapy.

Families understandably sometimes react badly to language such as, "The family is the problem." You can make the same point to a family in treatment by using language that conveys, "I think of your whole family as my client, rather than any one individual member of the family."

WHEN IS FAMILY THERAPY APPROPRIATE?

The primary criterion for deciding whether family therapy is an appropriate structure for treatment is a decision about the degree to which the adolescent client's problems result from family relationships and environment rather than from problems internal to the client. A second consideration is the degree to which the client is still involved with and influenced by the family. Sometimes problems that are primarily internal to the adolescent can be greatly helped by family participation, even when the family is not primarily the source of the problems. Third, it helps to have some sense of the potential for change within the family. It would make no sense to try family therapy to help an adolescent client if the family is currently embroiled in severe abuse, alcoholic violence, or psychosis.

Sholevar (1997) says that family therapy is clearly indicated when there are open and stressful conflicts among family members, even if none of the family members is showing symptoms of an emotional disorder. In addition, when one or more family members are exhibiting dysfunctional behavior, family therapy is often worth trying to identify subtle and covert family problems. Sholevar also points out that working with families of hospitalized adolescents is often effective, primarily when psychoeducational approaches are used.

Family therapy would be contraindicated in the case of extremely destructive behaviors in the family, as I mentioned earlier. It probably also should be avoided when one or more of the family members, probably the adolescent client, are unusually vulnerable, fragile, or recently hospitalized. The process of family therapy is complicated and sometimes stressful.

Also, in some cases you will have to make a judgment call based on your client's specific family situation. Depending on the setting in which you work, you will almost certainly have adolescent clients who will adamantly refuse to meet with their families. Often parents will refuse, sometimes angrily, to participate in family therapy because "the kid's the one with the problem. I'm not coming in there." Pitta (1995) notes that family members sometimes react with statements such as, "Fix my adolescent," "Don't trouble my marriage," "Don't expose my other children to therapy," "Let's keep therapy a secret. It's something to be ashamed of" (p. 100). In the face of this kind of resistance you often will have to find alternative modes of treatment.

Individual versus Family Therapy

Proponents of family therapy sometimes seem to be saying that a person in a relationship should always be treated along with the others involved in that relationship. In my opinion this is clearly an overstatement, especially in the treatment of adolescent clients. Family therapy is an important component of treating adolescents, most of whom are still intimately involved with their families, but if we could treat adolescents only in family therapy, we would eliminate most of what we do. There is a place for both approaches, but deciding when each is appropriate is difficult.

The ideal principle is that problems that result mainly from internal conflicts are best suited to individual therapy and that those that result from poor communication patterns and distorted relationships are best handled with multiple-client approaches, such as family therapy. In practice, though, nearly all problems have elements of both. In this case it is usually most effective to combine individual therapy and family therapy with adolescent clients.

GOALS OF FAMILY THERAPY

Setting goals in individual therapy is a complex enough process. In family therapy several individuals' best interests are involved, and these interests often conflict. Even the format in which clients are seen implies certain goals. Ideally, I say to all involved that my goal is that they all find the most satisfying solutions they can. But even before therapy starts, there is often a decision about whether an adolescent client's treatment will be primarily family therapy or primarily individual modes of treatment, with an occasional family session. Focusing on individual modes of treatment strongly implies a direction toward the adolescent's independence and autonomy, whereas focusing on family therapy means that the sought-after solutions can be found primarily in the family environment. The point is that family therapy nearly always involves complex and different specific goals. As with individual therapy, goals will emerge and change in the process of therapy as any one particular family works out its unique dynamics.

The specific goals of each family will be specific to their situation, of course, but it is worth discussing the general goals of family therapy. Sholevar (1997) lists four general goals: "(1) Explore family dynamics related to problems; (2) mobilize the family's internal strength and functional resources; (3) restructure the maladaptive interactional family styles; and (4) strengthen the family's problem-solving behavior" (p. 857). These goals are listed in roughly the order in which they occur in family therapy, and the rest of this chapter is designed to give you some tools for working toward these goals.

ASSESSMENT METHODS

There is some disagreement between family therapists who recommend conducting a standardized formal assessment of the family before planning a course of treatment and family therapists (who seem to be in the majority) who argue that it is almost impossible to separate the processes of assessing the family and treating the family. As Micucci (1998) says,

> In some approaches to therapy, assessment (or diagnosis) precedes intervention (treatment). In family therapy, the distinction between assessment and interventions is seen as an artificial one. A therapist assesses a family by carefully tracking how the family responds to his attempts to alter or modify their usual ways of relating to one another. (p. 7)

Similarly, Nichols (1999) says,

> Unlike some traditional approaches in which assessment and treatment could be separated into different stages or even into different endeavors in which one professional might meet with clients initially and a therapist be assigned subsequently, assessment and treatment are conducted simultaneously in family therapy from the beginning. Assessment is, of course, an ongoing process in which the therapist makes observations and interventions and subsequently changes his or her assessment and perceptions as feedback flows from the contract and interaction with the client system. (p. 141)

Formal assessment instruments for working with families have been shown to be useful in research studies (L'Abate & Bagarozzi, 1993; Miller et al., 1994; Beavers & Hampson, 1990). These measures can also be used in the clinical setting, but the information they yield tends to be more general and less specifically useful for guiding the therapist's interventions than are the therapist's ongoing observations.

One family assessment method that some therapists use is to have the family discuss and develop a genogram. Relationships among the family members and others in their life are diagrammed on a flip chart. Circles and squares with individuals' names in them are positioned to represent relative relationships, and lines of influence are drawn between the squares and circles. This process often gives both the therapist and the family members an overview of the current state of the family. Probably the most useful part of constructing a genogram is that the process leads to considerable discussion that the therapist then has a chance to observe.

TREATMENT METHODS

Relationships Are Still Primary but Are Much More Complicated

Nearly everybody who writes about family therapy stresses the importance of developing a good relationship with all family members who attend sessions. Minuchin (1974) has written extensively about the importance of joining with all members of the family within the first few minutes of every session. He kept time to notice and recognize each person, to check with them about each person's reactions to therapy sessions, to ask about personal concerns, and generally to establish an emotional connection with each person. A friend of mine who specializes in family therapy likes to say that her first job is to "win the family." This is no small task. In essence, joining involves a never-ending effort by the therapist to build a therapeutic alliance with every family member. One father, near the end of successful family therapy, said to the therapist, "I think the thing that made this work was that you were there for all of us." It had been an important lesson for him to see how the therapist could be there for him and for his adolescent son with whom he so often fought.

Swift (1993) says it well:

> The ultimate goal is to have a strong alliance with all family members in order to create an atmosphere of psychological safety in the sessions. Only in such a climate can growth and change occur. Inexperienced therapists are typically mesmerized by the power and prestige of the parents and inadvertently neglect children and adolescents in the family. While it is undoubtedly true that developing a treatment alliance with the parents is absolutely essential, one neglects the younger generation at considerable risk; often the way to the hearts and minds of the parents is through their children. (p. 382)

Different writers use different language with the same message. I will discuss Liddle's (1995) work in more detail later and see how he stresses the engagement process. Micucci (1998) talks about the ARCH of therapy: acceptance, respect, curiosity, and honesty. He says:

> The therapist makes a commitment to the relationship, and by holding the relationship in high esteem, he conveys to the other person the expectation that they also will hold the relationship with the therapist in high esteem. This is particularly important with adolescents, who often feel as if adults don't accept them, don't respect them, don't care what they think, and aren't honest with them. (p. 5)

Micucci also notes that "the most powerful resource for helping a person change is the relationships in which he or she participates. It's about as close as we get to an axiom in therapy that the quality of the therapeutic relationship is a key determinant of the success or failure of therapy" (p. 3). Here Micucci is talking about the nature and potential of family therapy. "Certainly I agree that our relationships with clients are critically important. But I'm talking here not only about the therapeutic relationship, but also about the healing potential of the natural relationships in a person's life" (Micucci, 1998, p. 3). In a sense, Micucci is presenting one of the strongest arguments in favor of family therapy. The relationship with a therapist can be important and influential, but it "is a means to an end, not an end in itself" (p. 4). The greatest good that a therapist can do is to help a client improve his or her relationships in everyday life, and the adolescent's family is potentially the source of relationships that will be healing in the long run. Micucci concludes that "the real healing takes place not in the therapeutic relationship but in the client's relationships with significant others" (p. 4).

Swift and Micucci are telling you that you have no power as a family therapist except the power you earn. No matter how clever you are, no family member has to listen to you or do what you say unless he or she wants to. First you must win the family.

Engaging the Adolescent, Engaging the Parents, Solving Problems

Liddle (1995) outlined a helpful approach to family treatment with adolescents that he calls multidimensional multisystems family therapy (MDFT). The strength of Liddle's approach is that it involves the many systems that impinge on the family, and it approaches problems from many directions. Liddle summarizes the philosophy of MDFT as

> We have a "Do what it takes" philosophy. This is not once-a-week, in-office therapy. Motivation is not assumed. It is the therapist's job to motivate family members. We do this by defining a core therapeutic task that helps each family member find a constructive, personally meaningful reason for coming. At the same time, we do not minimize the importance of service delivery components of treatment, such as where sessions are held or how transportation, babysitting, or other logistical matters affect attendance. (p. 51–52)

The actual treatment process of MDFT can be broken down into three general areas: (1) engaging the adolescent subsystem, (2) engaging the parental subsystem, and (3) engaging interaction between the parent and the adolescent. In other words, form a connection that motivates both the adolescent and the parents and then intervene in their process. Liddle is clear that interventions include both direct modifications of the way parents and the adolescent communicate and the involvement of all the systems involved with the family, including schools, probation officers, job agencies, and anything that fits "Do what it takes."

I use Liddle's general outline to explore these three general strategies. Obviously, much of what you have learned about forming a relationship with an adolescent will also apply here, and my discussion will draw from both Liddle's work and ideas from others, especially regarding specific interventions.

Engaging the Adolescent Subsystem

The adolescent client usually comes to therapy, and especially family therapy, with fairly negative expectations. From the adolescent's point of view, the whole setup looks as though the system (parents, professionals, and other assorted adults) is ganging up on the adolescent client. However, the therapist can behave in specific ways to change these expectations. Please review the information in chapter 2 about forming an alliance with an adolescent, especially in the first few minutes. You will need all of those skills in family therapy. You will not be neglecting the parents and will be motivating and engaging them, but your first job is usually to motivate and engage the adolescent, who will be thinking some version of, "What's in this for me?"

You must quickly make the adolescent feel understood in some way, perhaps even regarding his or her wish not to be in therapy. You also need to find some way to communicate that you are on the adolescent's side. This does not mean on his or her side against the parents; it means that you want something that will make the client's life better from his or her point of view. Parenthetically, it is worth saying that some clinicians do try to connect with an adolescent by implying, "I am on your side against your parents." This implication is a cheap shot that some people use because it often works in the short term; it often pleases adolescents and does win them over quickly. The problem, obviously, is that it alienates parents if they hear it, but it also usually carries a large cost even when they do not hear it directly from you. At some point adolescent clients are likely to throw it in a parent's face in a moment of anger: "My therapist said you're a lousy parent who never should have abandoned me by getting married again!" Even if this never happens, solutions to problems often involve working toward better relationships between parents and clients, and you will have worked against this process.

Liddle looks for a solid theme that comes from the adolescent that makes therapy make sense from the adolescent's point of view. Vague goals do not make sense to adolescents, and the goals of the parents or the school or the legal system are usually not the adolescent's goals. "It is critical to the engagement process to construct an individualized rationale for the therapy with each adolescent" (Liddle, 1995, p. 44). This is all another version of what I have stated so often about adolescent clients' need for structure. We are looking for a specific, well-defined goal that will motivate the adolescent to buy into the therapy process. An example that Liddle suggests is a plan to "see how you can learn to survive the streets" (p. 44). Other possibilities might include, "Eventually we might be able to write up some kind of contract with your parents where you could stay with the friends you like best but somehow they wouldn't worry about you so much" or "Can you and I figure out a list of four specific things you'd like changed and four you want to stay the way they are?"

The three most important elements of engaging an adolescent seem to be (1) making the adolescent feel understood and accepted, (2) helping the adolescent see that there is something to gain in the process, and (3) having a concrete, workable agenda that looks like a sensible way to proceed to the adolescent.

Engaging the Parental Subsystem

Sometimes the clinician has the luxury of being able to form an alliance with the adolescent client before seeing him or her with the family, but this is usually not the case. Normally, the family therapist's first contact is with the parents (or, often, just one parent) and the teenager. Occasionally, other siblings will attend this first session. As a family therapist, your job is to engage everyone in the treatment process, and it should be obvious that this will require every shred of clinical skill you have. Almost always, your first job is to engage the adolescent client, but you must do this in a way that does not alienate parents. This process is so complicated that it must be the primary focus of early sessions. Inexperienced family therapists are often eager to get to the nitty gritty of working on issues and fail to engage the family first. You may be tired of hearing this, but you have no power except the power you earn as a family therapist.

Before I discuss specific methods for engaging the parents, I need to stress the importance of therapist attitude (Colapinto, 1991; Liddle, 1995). In chapter 1 I discussed how some clinicians are able to work with adolescents and some seem incapable of it. Much of this difference is probably related to the clinician's conscious and unconscious belief system about teenagers and parents. Some clinicians tend to pathologize adolescents and their parents (Offer, Ostrov, & Howard, 1981). Many of these clinicians see even normal adolescents as caught up in turmoil and disorder (a myth I tried to counter in chapter 1) and have a tendency to think first, "What's wrong with this person?" This belief system makes it difficult to form an alliance and to engage adolescents and parents in treatment.

The alternative is not a blindly optimistic belief. The alternative is a belief—actually, it's more than a belief; it's an attitude that guides the clinician—that the parents and adolescent have the capacity to change and that, even now, they are trying to do the best that they can. This underlying attitude subtly influences the clinician's behavior in ways that communicate, "I'm in this together with you, and there are good things we can do together. Fundamentally, I trust you, and I understand that, as distressing as your situation is, it is not the result of your being bad people."

No matter how clever you are at hiding it, a pathology-oriented fundamental attitude subtly communicates, "There is something wrong with you people, and my job is to fix it." Parents and adolescents will respond with subtle and not-so-subtle resistance for reasons that neither they nor you will understand.

Finally, there is one aspect of therapist attitude that is a potential problem, especially among clinicians who feel themselves strongly drawn to work with adolescents. If the clinician holds a "blame the parents" attitude and sees the parents as the enemy against whom the adolescent and the clinician are comrades in battle, then family therapy will fail far more than it succeeds. In the previous section I talked about criticizing parents as a cheap-shot way to form an alliance with an adolescent. What I am talking about now is more subtle than that; I am talking about an underlying attitude of which the clinician may only be partially aware. If you like working with adolescents, you should at least think about this issue and perhaps find an understanding and accepting person with whom to talk it through.

The fundamental skill you need for engaging parents and adolescents in treatment at the same time is the same skill that I discussed with regard to group therapy in chapter 5: the ability to make several people feel understood at the same time, even when they disagree with each other. Family therapy is harder to do than group therapy, partly because the participants almost certainly disagree with each other more than clients in group therapy. I noted that your primary task is to engage the adolescent client with understanding, acceptance, motivation, and concrete planning. However, you cannot do this exclusively and ignore the parents while they sit there watching you interact with their son or daughter. The adolescent may be your primary focus, but you will also be tracking the parents' reactions and contributions and making them feel understood. It should be obvious that it is a bit of an artificial distinction to say that in this phase of treatment we are engaging the participants and in the next phase we will work on their patterns of interaction. All of your methods for making two or more people feel understood at the same time are both relationship builders and interventions in the process. As you articulate what a father is trying to say, you are both making the father feel understood and modeling good listening. The mother and the adolescent client cannot help but be affected by what you have done. You have taught by example and you have shown them a version of the father's message that they probably did not fully understand.

Liddle (1995) suggests that there "should be sensitivity to key dimensions of the current situation faced by the parent. For example, parents may be embarrassed about attending therapy, particularly in court-ordered treatment. . . . Sensitivity to previous unsuccessful attempts to obtain help is imperative" (p. 46). Some responses to the parents should communicate your assumption that they have been trying to do their best as parents and possibly to acknowledge that at least some of the problems are influenced by external events and things beyond their control. As with the adolescent client, you will need to find ways to make sense of the therapy process to the parents. There needs to be some discussion of how the concrete processes of therapy are intended to lead to specific outcomes.

In addition to being sensitive to the parents' expectation of being blamed for the problems, you should also listen for worry on their part that they will be expected to do most of the work and changing in fixing the problems. You can assure them that responsibility also lies with their son or daughter and that you will be working toward this end with the adolescent, perhaps even in separate individual sessions. As much as is realistic, the family's problems can be normalized by putting them in the context of normal adolescent development and the context of challenges and difficulties that other families face. Havas and Bonnar (1999) argue strongly that most family therapists do not take the social context of the family into account. This often results in the parents feeling blamed as the source of all problems and thus reluctant to discuss problems they face. "Work with families and adolescents must empower parents to recognize the sources of societal stress" (Havas & Bonnar, 1999, p. 121). Liddle (1995) also suggests that you communicate to the parents your belief that the adolescent's behavior is understandable and can change and that it is essential that the parents be involved in the change process.

Especially early in treatment, the therapist communicates, implicitly and explicitly, "I really want to hear your story" to everyone in the family. This takes time and sensitivity both to the painful emotions and to the hopeful, positive things that people try to say.

Focusing on Interactions and Looking for Solutions

Once you have established good relationships and have engaged the family in treatment, you can use a wide variety of techniques and interventions. These methods can be understood in two large areas. First, understanding, facilitating, and changing communication patterns is essential for therapy to have a long-lasting effect; second, the family will have specific problems that will call for specific solutions. Your goal is to help the family deal with their present problems, but it is also to provide them with the tools to deal with new problems in the future.

It is useful to think in terms of "the family is the client," and so we are working toward change both within the individuals and in the interactions between them. The first focus in family therapy is on facilitating communication between the parents and the adolescent and between the parents. This is done primarily through modeling of good communication by the therapist, making suggestions about specific interactions in the session, commenting on patterns of interaction that the therapist perceives, and sometimes direct teaching of communication skills.

It is also important to remember that relationship building and engagement are continuous processes that go on throughout treatment. Techniques are always presented within the therapeutic attitude.

Modeling Good Listening   You will use all your skills at hearing both the cognitive and emotional meaning of what one of the family members is saying, and, as you communicate that understanding to the person, you will also be sensitive to its impact on others in the room. You might say to the mother, "It sounds to me like you have mixed feelings about how mad Heather is that you searched her room. I think you were desperate about your worry that she was using cocaine, but you also felt guilty about doing it. Is that pretty close?" Assuming that the mother confirms the accuracy of this comment, you might then turn to Heather and ask, "Did you know that she felt both of those things?" This interchange accomplishes several purposes. It makes the mother feel understood, and it articulates her thoughts and feelings in a way that she intended but may never have articulated herself. This is likely to reward and motivate the mother for sharing more. Turning to the daughter this way engages her in understanding her mother (through the therapist as an intermediary) in a way that she probably had not understood her mother before and in a way that almost certainly interrupted their older ways of interacting. In this scenario it is likely that the therapist has already observed the mother and the daughter interacting solely with anger, accusations, and name calling. To complicate matters, of course, you will also be tracking the impact of this interchange on the father, sensing such issues as does he seem to take sides, does he understand the mother's concerns, and how does he react to the issue of searching his daughter's room?

Direct Interventions in Communication Patterns   Sometimes it is helpful to directly intervene in communication patterns. You may notice that the father tends to answer all questions, even when they are directed at other family members. Or you may notice a destructive interaction pattern in which family members set up straw men by exaggerating what another person has said in a way that makes it unreasonable. For example, the son might say, "I need to have some friends." A straw man response might be, "You just can't spend all your time with friends and flunk out of school."

Of course, there are hundreds of possible communication patterns that might call for intervention, and you have several tools available for these interventions. One method that both interrupts the destructive interaction patterns and forces some listening is to ask the parent to put into words what the son meant, speaking as though the parent were the son. The first time you try this, the person will likely struggle because he or she really did not listen to what was said. In this case it is probably best to let the person off the hook by saying something such as, "Well, let me tell you what I thought he was saying, and then we will check with him to see if I'm right. I thought he meant something like 'I at least need to have some friends, but I but I don't mean that they would take up my whole life.'" This might be sufficient as an intervention, or you might go on to explain and describe the general communication patterns of exaggerating what the other person said in a way that distorts it.

Verbal Methods vs. Action Methods   Guldner (1990) reported a study with interesting implications for doing family therapy. He studied 24 families who received structural family therapy (Minuchin, 1974). Half of the families received treatment that was primarily verbal and half received action methods. In structural family therapy one of the therapist's most important jobs is to identify patterns of interaction in a family that are causing problems. The therapist observes the family's style as members respond to questions and interact in discussions. One primary technique the therapist then uses is to set up an enactment in which the family re-creates and plays out a situation typical of their interactions at home. Most structural family therapists carry out enactments only through verbal recreations of the situation. Guldner was trained both in structural family therapy and in psychodrama, and he has combined the two approaches into an action-based method. Family members reenact typical scenes with movement and dialogue. He reports that this is "a form of therapy that I find works especially well with adolescents involved in family therapy. Generally, adolescents are less comfortable with verbal communication than they are with activity. Through the use of action methods during the therapy process, they tend to feel less 'one-down' from the adults" (Guldner, 1990, p. 143).

Some of the more interesting methods used in this action-oriented approach to family therapy are sculpting, role playing, and psychodrama.

In sculpting family members take turns arranging people into scenes that represent different situations. There are endless possibilities, of course, but the therapist might ask the adolescent to set up the scene for "when an argument is about to start" or "when Mom and Dad are on the same side against the kids." Then this sculpted scene forms the basis for discussion. For example, power imbalances and boundaries within the family are often revealed by sculpting.

In role playing a specific conversation or situation might be acted out. Sometimes, family members will take someone else's role. For example, the father is asked to play out how the adolescent should talk to his mother. This is usually not easy and forces the father and the whole family to think through what specific behaviors are effective and ineffective.

Psychodrama resembles role playing, but it is more complicated and usually involves the development of a story line that the members act out, again sometimes taking on other people's roles. The therapist often participates in and discusses the process of developing the story.

Guldner was cautious in claiming results that could be generalized to family therapy in general, but there were a number of areas in which the action-oriented therapy seemed to be more well received by the families in treatment, especially with regard to the participation and involvement of the adolescent members of the families.

Look for the Family's Strengths: The Family Is the Problem Solver Almost every family has made some attempts to solve their problems. Almost every family has strengths that could be mobilized in the search for new solutions. Most of the techniques I have discussed so far have focused on identifying and changing destructive interaction patterns. The danger is that the family therapist will focus so much on what is wrong that potential new solutions will be missed. Families who enter treatment are normally so caught up in conflicts, problems, and pathology that they often also focus on how things are going wrong rather than how they could do better or even on the parts of their current family functioning that are already positive and constructive. We all selectively perceive what we expect to see, and clinicians who are pathologizers will miss many of the family's problem-solving attempts. Attune yourself to hear strengths, to hear problem solving that has worked in the past, and to hear good intentions among the many negative issues that come up.

Looking for the family's strengths will require you to do more sitting back and listening than many therapists do. Rushing in with your solutions often will interfere both with the family's attempts to come up with solutions on their own and with your opportunity to hear about strengths and things that are going well. The greatest gift you will give the family is the opportunity to solve their own problems.

Behavioral Methods   The application of behavioral approaches to family therapy is, of course, based on the principles of learning I discussed in chapter 4. A behaviorally oriented family therapist also focuses on making a good connection with the family and tends to think in terms of reinforcement and punishment. The therapist, for example, would be interested in what kinds of reinforcers maintain maladaptive behaviors and maladaptive communication patterns in the family. In general, the therapist discourages punitive ways that the family interacts with each other and helps the family learn new problem-solving skills based on reinforcement principles.

As we also saw in chapter 4, modern behavior therapy looks at both overt behaviors and patterns of thinking and cognition. Behavior therapists draw from many different resources, such as parent-training programs and communication skills programs. Behavioral family therapists are more likely than other therapists to encourage the family to make explicit behavioral contracts based on the principles of reinforcement and behavioral exchange between family members.

It is misleading, of course, to imply that these principles of learning and methods are used only by people who refer to themselves as behavior therapists. The principles of learning can provide both the therapist and the family with deeper understanding of the causes of family behaviors, and virtually all approaches acknowledge the influence of reinforcement. For example, many family therapists have observed the family pattern in which the adolescent son or daughter exhibits symptoms of emotional disturbance for no apparent reason. Careful observation then reveals that the parents have serious relationship problems between themselves, but these problems do not surface when the parents are mutually focused on the teenager's illness. A behavioral analysis would say that the teenager was being reinforced for being ill by the powerful effects of anxiety reduction that comes from the temporary elimination of parental conflict. This would be an example of negative reinforcement—the reward of escaping something painful.

Psychoeducational Approaches   Psychoeducational interventions with families are probably most commonly used when the adolescent client is suffering from a major mental illness, such as clinical depression or schizophrenia (Sholevar, 1997). Sessions are based less on discussion of and interventions in family dynamics and more on delivering information that is designed to help the family cope with the young person's disorder. The focus of treatment is highly structured and often centers on concrete actions, such as finding community resources, crisis management, and housing arrangements. Psychoeducational sessions also include some opportunity for the family to ask questions and discuss issues, but more exploratory kinds of family therapy are usually delayed until the patient and the family have reached some equilibrium in their adjustment to the disorder.

Combining Individual Sessions with Family Sessions   As noted earlier, some family therapists insist that all treatment should involve the whole family and that it is counterproductive to see individual family members in sessions. This is usually based on a strong belief in systems theory. Many family therapists, however, take the more pragmatic view that there can be advantages to meeting individually with family members (Liddle, 1995; Micucci, 1998;

Pitta, 1995). In any case the treatment of adolescents often is centered on the individual teenage client, and family therapy is one piece of the larger treatment program. Especially if the young person is being treated in a treatment center or hospital, either on an outpatient or an inpatient basis, family therapy is usually not the primary focus.

Individual sessions are sometimes helpful to prepare adolescents or parents to make better use of the family therapy sessions. This preparation can include teaching about the nature of family therapy without being caught up in the complex dynamics of a family therapy session. They can be an opportunity for a client to rehearse different ways of interacting with other family members in role playing with the individual therapist. Family therapy sessions are so strongly oriented around problem-based patterns of interaction that specific content issues sometimes are difficult to deal with in depth. Both parents and adolescents often say things in individual sessions that they are reluctant to bring up in a family session. These might, of course, involve secrets, but they also might involve sensitive issues that need to be discussed but that would bring up so much emotion in a family session that they would never be discussed. One serious problem with family therapy is that, for all the advantages of seeing family members together, there are many things people just will not say in the presence of other family members, especially early in treatment. There are issues of mistrust and unwillingness to become vulnerable by giving the other person ammunition. There is no easy solution to this problem. With families there is the risk that seeing just one person in individual sessions might help make that person the identified patient and set up a special status that breeds mistrust of the therapist and other members of the family. Depending on how central family therapy is to treatment, you need to communicate that the family is your client, that your goal is to help them establish solutions as a family, but that you will occasionally see individual members. If there are co-therapists, it is important that each therapist see each client, so that neither therapist becomes identified as on the side of one or two family members. The ground rules for the sessions are tricky and therefore must be made absolutely clear. I usually say, "The purpose of the sessions is that sometimes there are things that are hard to say in front of other family members, especially at first. If you want things kept private from the individual sessions, you can say so, and I will respect that. Whether we deal with those things eventually in family sessions will be up to you." This requires the therapist to have a good memory and carries some clear risks, but my experience has been that such sessions are especially helpful early in therapy and that they actually facilitate the family's dealing with threatening issues more quickly. The issues often would never come up just in family sessions, but trying them out in individual sessions helps make them more manageable.

BRIEF FAMILY THERAPY

In chapter 3 I introduced the principles of brief therapy with individual adolescents. In essence, I said that the three key principles are (1) to develop a good therapeutic alliance, (2) to establish a fairly clear focus for the treatment rather than thinking in terms of wide-ranging exploration, and (3) to think in terms of specific, modest goals that are within reach (Swift, 1993). The same general principles apply to brief family therapy with a few additional guidelines: (1) Establish a good relationship with all family members, (2) work on communication skills, (3) examine the family's currently unsuccessful solutions to problems, and (4) examine patterns of interaction that cause trouble for the family.

First, the focus is almost by necessity on interpersonal relationships. Of course it is important to establish a good connection with all family members, especially the adolescent. In longer term treatment, however, the relationship between the therapist and the family members is itself often a source of important healing. In general, though, brief therapy does not give time for such a powerful bond to form with the therapist. The emphasis, therefore, should be more on the relationships among family members. As Swift (1993) says, "The emphasis in brief family therapy is on releasing latent healing power within the family itself" (p. 381).

The second focus is to create a structured and fairly well-ordered process in which to focus on communication skills. Sometimes, creating this necessary order requires the therapist to be a referee who interrupts disruptive communication patterns. The therapist might use such a moment to do some direct teaching of how confrontations should focus on behaviors rather than on personalities and name calling. Swift (1993) actually keeps a soccer whistle in his desk that he uses for extremely disruptive families. Most family therapists seem to use the term "referee" to describe part of their role to families, but Swift's whistle certainly brings the principle to life. In addition to the "confront behavior only" principle, one of the most important communication skills a family must learn is to listen to each other. In general, people do not listen to each other very well, and families in treatment are worse than most.

Because treatment will be so brief, the therapist often must use some direct interventions, such as saying, "I don't see how you people are ever going to make this family work if you don't start listening to each other." Then the therapist will probably have to more gently illustrate this statement with examples and with moving back to making the family members feel understood. The therapist might say, "I think each of you feels pretty threatened by what other people say here, so it's understandable that it's hard to listen. But this is really important. Here's what I thought happened a minute ago. I think Dad and Robert both made important, valid points but neither of you heard what the other one was saying. I thought Dad was telling Robert something like, 'I really hate it when you take the car, even for short trips, without asking.' Robert, it sounded like you took that to mean something like, 'You're so irresponsible, so you can't use the car.' Is that what it sounded like? I really don't think that's what he meant, and I'm sure it's not what he said. But then, Dad, when Robert said he needed the car sometimes, I think you took it that he was saying he wanted to use it just to party, so of course you reacted negatively. My point is that unless I can help you listen to each other better, we're not going to get very far." The therapist—you—probably will not have time to say all of this at once, but it illustrates the principle.

Third, the family will have tried various ways to deal with their problems and especially with their adolescent's problems. It is important to discuss these attempts at solutions to examine how they might be contributing to the problem. If the adolescent is afraid to leave home, the parents might have, in frustration, started yelling at her in an attempt to motivate her. Or they might be criticizing her for not doing more during the few times she does get out of the house. Some of the family's coping methods might actually be helpful, but many will not be. This period of discussion will be aimed at sorting out which solutions work and which do not.

Fourth, patterns of interaction can have a life of their own in families. In some families, for example, each member has come to expect criticism and therefore reacts to nearly any interaction with hostility and criticism. The vicious circle that gets set up can continue for years. The therapist observes interaction patterns in the therapy session and listens to reports of incidents from the family's life in order to identify these patterns.

The trick in brief family therapy is to find a limited focus and to have small, achievable goals.

FAMILY THERAPY IS THE MOST COMPLICATED TREATMENT FORMAT

Most therapists find family therapy to be the most complex and difficult form of treatment. Therapists need all of their individual therapy skills, all of their ability to track interactions, as in group therapy, and a deep understanding of family dynamics. In addition, the clinician's own issues around family both inform and distort the treatment process. Cultural issues are especially sensitive in family therapy because the norms for family structure and behaviors vary so widely among cultures. It is especially difficult to treat families from cultures with which you are not intimately familiar. As with other treatment formats, you may find your special niche in family therapy, and you will discover this only through experience.

Recommended Reading

Beavers, W. R., & Hampson, R. B. (1990). *Successful families: Assessment and intervention.* New York: Norton.

L'Abate, L., & Bagarozzi, D. A. (1993). *Sourcebook of marriage and family evaluation.* New York: Brunner/Mazel.

Micucci, J. A. (1998). *The adolescent in family therapy.* New York: Guilford Press.

TREATMENT OF SPECIFIC DISORDERS

We are not sophisticated enough yet in our knowledge to diagnose a highly specific emotional disorder and then assign a highly specific treatment, but we can make some diagnostic decisions that will influence how we deal with a specific adolescent. In the first section of this chapter I look at some of the valid uses of the diagnostic process and some of the dangers at our current level of knowledge. Then I briefly discuss some of the special treatment considerations for a few different disorders.

This chapter is not a textbook on abnormal psychology, and I do not describe different disorders with the goal of teaching you to diagnose them. You should familiarize yourself with the process of assessment and diagnosis through courses and books designed for that purpose. The purpose of this chapter is to give you practical advice about a few of the treatment situations you will encounter, especially those situations with special circumstances. This chapter is selective, and I have tried to anticipate the situations that might cause you trouble and the situations where special circumstances call for special attention.

SOME COMMENTS
ON ASSESSMENT AND DIAGNOSIS

Assessment and diagnosis are generally seen as essential parts of the treatment of adolescents. This is especially true in clinics and hospitals, where some process of assessment is almost always the initial stage of a treatment program. In private practice assessment is more likely to be treated as an ongoing process that is part of treatment itself, unless the young person has been specifically referred for an assessment. Ideally, clinical practice would consist of an accurate assessment that leads directly to the application of specific treatments. In real life, however, the process is much messier and less defined than the ideal. For example, many adolescents receive multiple diagnoses over the course of a few years, many of which contradict each other. Our assessment methods are not as valid and reliable as they should be, but it is clear that we must make the best assessments we can because the judgments that come out of our assessments have life-changing consequences for our clients.

First, I am going to try to upset you by saying that you will face many troubling dilemmas over assessment, but you also must do the best you can with the tools we have. After I have you upset and worried, I will discuss positive aspects of the assessment process. Assessments are necessary, but they need to be treated with respectful caution. They also need to be presented to clients with tentative caution. Diagnoses have a powerful labeling effect, in which clients *become* their label in the minds of others and themselves. Young people often misunderstand the limits of diagnoses, and you may be distressed to have one tell you, "I just found what I am. I'm an obsessive-compulsive." The label has a power to become a reality that is hard for the client to escape. I have been working with adolescents for many years and have been troubled by the dilemmas presented by the assessment process ever since I was an intern. I can remember the frustration of a fellow intern who used to proclaim, "The best way to predict a kid's diagnosis is to know the name of his psychiatrist." He was exaggerating the case, but the process of assessment and diagnosis is sometimes capricious. Some years later, I found a kind of bittersweet comfort in knowing that I was not alone in my experience when I read a chapter by Garfield (1986) in which he made an observation that most practicing clinicians will recognize as true: "Anyone who has worked in a large clinical setting has probably noticed that there is no unanimity among the staff in diagnostic conferences. I have participated in staff conferences in which the final decision [on a patient's diagnosis] was conclusively settled by an eight to seven vote of the staff members present" (p. 101).

Garfield's complaint was with the process of deciding on a diagnosis, but reaching a formal diagnosis is only one part of the broader process of assessment. It is important that we see assessment as a multifaceted process that draws information from many sources. The assessment process is centered on the assessment questions. It is not unusual to receive an assessment referral that says something to the effect of, "Please assess this young man." This referral should be sent back with the question, "What do you want to know about him?" We are not just being difficult when we ask this question; we are asking for the assessment questions. Examples of assessment questions are, "Is this boy's difficulty in school the result of low intelligence, a learning disorder, emotional interference with learning, or some other cause?" This is a more meaningful request than, "Please assess him," because the information and requested decision structure the nature of the assessment. In general, the assessment process starts with a description of the troublesome behaviors, tries to understand the causes of the behaviors, and results in recommendations for changing those causes.

ASSESSMENT AS PART OF TREATMENT VERSUS ASSESSMENT TO ESTABLISH A DIAGNOSIS

Assessment is a broad-ranging process that draws from many sources. Establishing a formal diagnosis is one part of assessment in which clinicians assign a label for the category of problem a client has. Establishing a diagnosis is almost always done from a perspective outside the client. The process is analogous to establishing a medical diagnosis during which the patient is consulted but an outside expert makes a decision about a label or category. The assessment process can be and often is also carried out from this perspective. One of the realities of working in the era of managed care is that the system often demands this kind of formal diagnosis. It is often useful, however, to see assessment as an ongoing process that is seamlessly integrated with the treatment process.

Many assessments and diagnoses of adolescents are done at one point in time and are based on relatively brief contact with the client. Two problems with this practice are, first, that adolescent behavior and emotion can be erratic and labile and therefore might be quite different if the assessment were done at a different time and, second, that the nature of emotional problems is that many of their causes are not consciously perceivable by either the client or the assessor. It is wise to treat any assessment as a tentative approximation of an individual client and to think of assessment as an emerging process. As the treatment progresses, both the client and the clinician will see different aspects of the client's problems and, perhaps more important, will make new discoveries about the client. In other words, the assessment will emerge and change.

Different Professions Bring Different Perspectives

Although the tools of different professions overlap, one of the most valuable aspects of being part of a clinical treatment team is that each profession brings with it a special expertise in assessing specific areas of a client's functioning. The occupational therapist might pick up psychomotor problems that the psychologist's tests could miss. A social worker is primed to notice environmental causes more than a psychiatrist, who might be more focused on internal and physiological factors. Assessment of adolescents is a complex process that needs these different perspectives, and it is a good idea for members of each profession to be receptive to input from other professions. Each of us will be taught a different set of tools, and we need to be aware of both the strengths and the limitations of our tools.

VALID USES OF ASSESSMENT AND DIAGNOSIS

Although there are clearly problems with the diagnostic process, there is also evidence that we can validly and reliably make many diagnoses, especially among the major kinds of disorders, and these decisions do have an impact on treatment. Schizophrenic disorders, for example, almost always require some medical intervention. Bipolar depression, as another example, requires a different approach than depression that results from tragic loss. We need to use assessment and diagnosis and to continue to develop more valid systems, but we need to use them cautiously and only in conjunction with many sources of information as we go about our work of treating adolescents.

ANXIETY, MOOD, AND EATING DISORDERS

In the past the problems discussed in this section probably would have been called neurotic problems. They are severe problems in living that do not involve a significant loss of contact with reality. Some of these problems may involve physiological causes, but they are also significantly caused by the individual's past experiences. The term *neurosis* has fallen out of favor because it seemed to imply that these problems are illnesses, when they are better understood as *problems in living*.

It is extremely important to remember that, if these are problems in living and not illnesses, trying to categorize and label these problems carries both advantages and risks. Most of the adolescent clients you see will not fit cleanly into a diagnostic category. Some will, of course, but most will sometimes seem depressed and at other times a bit compulsive and maybe even phobically fearful at other times.

Anxiety Disorders

Many kinds of anxiety disorders have been described in the literature on diagnosing adults. However, although we can reliably and validly make a general diagnosis of anxiety disorder in adolescents, attempts to diagnose specific kinds of anxiety disorders are "limited by poor discriminant validity and lack of sensitivity to developmental levels" (Schniering, Hudson, & Rapee, 2000, p. 453). Most of what I have discussed in this book has fitted most closely the treatment of adolescent problems that center around anxiety, fear, insecurity, and other painful emotions. Therefore I will not spend much time in this chapter on special treatment considerations.

The most important point to be made here is that we should think of anxiety disorders among adolescent clients as a large, general category, and treatment should be guided by the unique nature of each client's problems. We need to ask the individual client about his or her anxiety without worrying about categorizing it. As Schniering, Hudson, and Rapee (2000) say, "It is critical to obtain information from children about their own anxiety, in addition to reports from other informants" (p. 473).

Affective Disorders: Suicide and Depression

The excessive sadness of depression is so distressing to people in the adolescent's life and it is so common that you will likely see many depressed young people in treatment. As with anxiety disorders, much of what I have already discussed applies strongly to affective disorders.

Special Treatment Issues   Treatment of affective disorders falls into two categories: medical treatments and psychological treatments.

In general, medications are a bigger issue in treating depression than in treating anxiety. Antidepressant medications are widely used in the treatment of depressive disorder in adults, and approximately 70% improve with medications, which is approximately the same percentage that improves with various forms of psychotherapy (Weiner, 1992). Weiner suggests that some combination of medications and therapy is worth trying with adolescent clients with unipolar depression, but Lock (1996) says,

> As a child and adolescent psychiatrist, I am often asked to evaluate a depressed teenager for a medication trial of antidepressants. I always begin such evaluations by having a frank discussion with the referring clinician, the family, and the teenager about our limited knowledge of antidepressant use in teenagers. I tell them that a variety of such medications have been tried in adolescents. Those that have been most carefully studied have not been shown to be more efficacious than placebo medications. (p. 168)

Lock goes on to say, "In terms of medications, bipolar disorder is one of the more treatable of psychiatric disorders, even among adolescents. In fact, unlike psychopharmacology as a treatment for major depression or dysthymia, it appears that adolescent onset and adult onset bipolar disorders have similar response rates to medication" (pp. 169–170). Both Lock and Weiner say that medication is especially important in the treatment of the mania of bipolar disorder.

Weiner (1992) notes that "an extensive literature demonstrates the effectiveness of many types of psychotherapy in treating affective disorder, including psychodynamic, behavioral, cognitive, and interpersonal approaches" (p. 145). The most widely researched approach to treatment of adolescent depression is cognitive behavioral therapy (CBT), as I discussed in chapter 4 (Lewinsohn & Clarke, 1999; Sommers-Flanagan and Sommers-Flanagan, 1997). In fact, depressed adolescents seem to react especially well to CBT early in treatment. It is often reassuring to have relatively structured activities that can have a relatively quick impact on the adolescent's depressed mood. Often this initial relief of sadness is all that is involved in treatment, but as treatment continues, it is usually helpful to go beyond the initial application of CBT methods to more insight-oriented methods.

Weiner (1992) argues that ultimately, the treatment of adolescent depression must deal with the client's sense of loss. In addition, he notes that it is especially important in treating adolescent depression to think in terms of helping to change and manipulate the client's environment in ways that diminish the sense of loss by minimizing disappointment and increasing gratification through the client's participation in activities that bring both positive emotions and a sense of accomplishment.

Adolescent Suicide   Treating affective disorders in adolescents always requires a kind of quiet vigilance about the issue of suicide. Suicide is the third leading cause of death for people under age 18, and the rate of adolescent suicide has been rising. Nearly all therapists with whom I have discussed suicide find it one of the most difficult issues they have to deal with, especially with adolescent clients. When the therapist has been involved in the very issues of emotional distress that contribute to suicide, thoughts over what might have been done that wasn't are difficult to resolve. Therapists' trouble in dealing with suicide makes this a special area of deafness in hearing clients. Intuitively, it often seems to the therapist that talking about suicide might make the risk greater, and so clues are missed or intentionally avoided. Your client might say, "I'm not sure it's all worth it, but at least I know there's one way to find peace." Because this statement may or may not refer to suicide, you do not want to suggest death in a way that might be frightening to the client. He or she might have been talking about some other way to find peace, but you cannot ignore the possibility that the implicit topic is suicide. You might firmly but gently get ahead of this client without using the word *suicide*. "I'm not sure of all you mean there, but sometimes you'd like to give up—to stop this pain by escaping it somehow. How? Just by stopping everything?" This response is forthright but not unduly frightening and will probably elicit further discussion that will clarify the suicide issue.

If there is any hint that concerns you about suicide, you should pursue the possibility both through gentle exploration and sometimes through direct questioning. Obviously, if there is reason to suspect that the teenager is actively suicidal and has a plan to carry out his or her intentions, you must intervene through hospitalization or some other direct action. Most of your contacts, however, will be less clearly dangerous, and you will want to develop the art of negotiating contracts with adolescents about suicidal behavior. These contracts are a vehicle for discussing suicide forthrightly and constructively, and they seem to have an effective preventive role.

I might, for example, negotiate an agreement that if the client starts to think seriously about suicide, he or she agrees to call me and set up an appointment immediately, or to phone a suicide hotline (whose number we memorize together).

As soon as a therapist is sure that a client is hinting at suicide, the therapist does a great service by using explicit words to give the client freedom to discuss the real issue. It is frightening to talk so openly about suicide, but you really have no choice. Ignoring the issue will not make suicide not seem peaceful to the client. It is unlikely that you can argue or persuade the person out of the feelings. You can explore the feelings together. In the process of this exploring, you might express some of your own feelings and reactions, saying something such as, "You probably know this, but I want to say that it matters to me that you live." If done sensitively, this would be an expression of concern and caring, not a judgmental guilt message that the client shouldn't feel the way he or she does.

Suicide talk should always be taken seriously and dealt with openly. It is sometimes used manipulatively by clients, especially when dependency is a central issue, and thus you will have to walk a narrow line between refusing to deal with the issue and being upset and overly responsive to the implicit threat that if you do not give your client more, you will have the client's life on your conscience.

Eating Disorders

The treatment of eating disorders in adolescents is especially challenging and potentially especially rewarding. On one hand, these disorders can be frighteningly destructive and even life-threatening, and their grip on clients can be so insidious and powerful that the clinician often feels at war with a vicious opponent, battling for the health of the client. On the other hand, early intervention is crucial to a successful outcome, and adolescence is often the starting point for eating disorders. For this reason I pay extra attention to some issues that clinicians often find useful in recognizing and treating eating disorders. One reason for you to be familiar with the signs of eating disorders is that you can have a preventive influence with young people who may be experimenting with intentional vomiting or laxatives as a way to lose weight. It is especially important that clinicians are aware of some significant differences between adult eating disorders and adolescent eating disorders. As we will see, these differences influence the diagnosis and treatment process with adolescent clients.

What an Eating Disorder Feels Like   It is difficult for a person who does not have an eating disorder to understand the compelling intensity of what feels like a cruel judge that seems to be a part of the client but over which the client feels no control. The essence of experiencing this judge is that being fat is overwhelmingly *wrong*. It feels morally wrong; the person feels horrible and worthless, with a worthlessness so deep that only words such as *evil* seem sufficient to describe it. Clients often describe it as though there is a voice constantly nagging and berating them.

This revulsion for being fat is combined with a distorted body image so that the person feels fat at almost any weight. Having *any* fat feels wrong, so the client almost continuously feels horrible, lazy, worthless, and evil, and the only temporary escape from this unbearable pain about the self comes from aggressive attempts to lose more weight. A principle that I have discussed many times in this book is that anxiety reduction is an extremely powerful reinforcer. The anxiety that drives eating disorders is so intense that anything that reduces it is extremely difficult to resist; the immediate moments of relief, even though temporary, are far more compelling even than the knowledge that extreme weight loss can, and sometimes does, kill people.

Bulimia Nervosa and Anorexia Nervosa   Anorexia and bulimia are similar disorders in that they both are characterized by a morbid fear of gaining weight and of losing control over eating behavior. The most obvious difference between them is that anorexia results in extreme thinness, but bulimia often does not. Most people with bulimia are within 10% of their normal weight, but people with anorexia are so dramatically skinny that their lives are often at risk.

Bulimia is more common than anorexia, and bulimia is characterized primarily by binging. The person eats a large amount of food, usually junk food, in a way that feels out of the person's control. Thus bulimia is defined both by the amount of food eaten at one time and the experience of being compelled to binge, even though the person would rather not. Because this out of control binging threatens the person with weight gain, which is totally unacceptable, bulimia also involves various strategies to compensate for the binge eating and to prevent weight gain.

The most common strategy is to use purging techniques to get rid of the excess food; about two-thirds of people with bulimia use purging strategies (Hsu, 1990).

DSM-IVTR differentiates between purging type and nonpurging type bulimia. Purging techniques can include self-induced vomiting immediately after a binge, the use of laxatives, and the use of diuretics. The vomiting usually is accomplished by sticking a finger down the throat to trigger the gag reflex. These methods are not very effective. Even immediate vomiting gets rid of only about half of the calories consumed; laxatives have little effect because they work so long after the binge, and diuretics have virtually no effect because they rid the body only of water, which will be replaced almost immediately. None of this matters to the client with bulimia, however, because he or she is desperate to get rid of the calories consumed. Terms you often hear in clinical settings include binging and purging and the binge/purging cycle.

Other than purging techniques the most common strategies used to undo the effects of a binge are extensive fasting between binges and excessive exercise.

A number of serious medical consequences are associated with bulimia, especially when purging is used. Repeated vomiting often erodes the enamel on a person's teeth, and it can cause a chubby facial appearance because it causes enlargement of the salivary glands. In addition, the loss of electrolytes can cause cardiac arrhythmia and kidney failure. Many deaths attributable to bulimia are the result of these two problems.

In contrast to bulimia, anorexia is marked by extremely successful attempts at caloric restriction and dramatic weight loss that often leave the person looking skeletal. Another important difference is that people with bulimia often feel ashamed of their problem and deeply distressed by their lack of control over eating behavior, whereas people with anorexia are often proud of what they perceive as their highly disciplined eating behavior. Anorexia is at the same time less common and a more severe disorder than bulimia.

One kind of anorexia is similar to bulimia and is called the binge eating/purging type. The difference is that the person with anorexia "binges" on much smaller amounts of food and purging is more consistent. In general, with anorexia purging that involves frequent use of laxatives is associated with a longer duration of the disorder (Turner et al., 2000). The other major subtype of anorexia is called the restricting type, in which the person goes to great lengths to avoid taking in food. Although the word *anorexia* actually means loss of appetite, this is not quite accurate; people with anorexia often feel intense hunger, and it is often these feelings of hunger that most strongly awaken the harsh internal judge that demands that the person restrict eating. Enduring the hunger, however, is far easier than enduring the harsh self-judgments that would result from giving in to hunger.

It is almost impossible for an adolescent with anorexia to be thin enough. Any small weight gain, or even staying the same weight from one day to the next, can throw the young person into a state of anxiety or depression. Only weight loss satisfies the voice of the anorexia, and the young person truly believes that she is disgustingly overweight. Seeing herself in the mirror is upsetting because the person in the mirror is perceived as too fat. This self-misperception is one of the most important reasons that anorexia is difficult to treat. The client does not believe that there is any problem except that she is too fat. In most cases the young person is brought into treatment by someone else, and one of the most difficult and important steps in treating her is to engage her in a treatment alliance in which both the client and the therapist are working toward the same goals.

In addition to the obvious problem of starvation, the medical complications of anorexia include the stopping of menstruation, dry skin, extreme sensitivity to cold, and possibly low heart rate and blood pressure. As with bulimia, if the person induces vomiting frequently, the loss of electrolytes can result in heart and kidney problems.

Signs of Eating Disorders   In the next section I discuss formal criteria for diagnosing eating disorders, but in this section I need to examine warning signs that the clinician should be aware of on a day-to-day basis. We do not want to hover intrusively in our clients' lives, but we do need to be sensitive to the possibility of eating disorders. Intensive early treatment of eating disorders can prevent many of the severe physical consequences, and long-term positive outcomes are much more likely when treatment starts near the onset of these problems. Unhealthy eating is practically an identifying characteristic of adolescence in our culture, but this is different from unhealthy attempts at weight control and, probably more important, obsessive thinking about weight, eating, exercise, and body shape. These are not certain indications of an eating disorder; rather, they are just reasons for the clinician to be alert.

Often a young person is enormously ambivalent about seeking help for eating problems. Adamant denial that there is a problem with eating can coexist with the adolescent's feeling that something is wrong. Many clinicians report that adolescent clients often seek help for other problems but that a sensitive listener can pick up hints of concerns about eating in an assessment interview or during the therapy (Sanders, 1996).

Woodside (1995) described five potential danger signs to help clinicians distinguish ordinary dieting from dieting that might suggest a potential eating disorder:

1. Decreasing weight goals are characteristic of an adolescent at risk for anorexia. Most teenagers on a diet are pleased when they reach their weight goal, but the young person at risk is never satisfied with reaching one goal; she needs to keep setting lower and lower weight goals.

2. Most normal adolescent dieters react to weight loss with an increased sense of satisfaction with their bodies, but the person at risk often reacts to weight loss with what seems like a paradoxical increase in self-criticism of the body. This increasing self-criticism can be a worrisome sign of body image distortions.

3. Most adolescents increase their social contacts when they lose weight, but a warning sign for eating disorders is when weight loss is followed by increasing social isolation and a marked increase in focus on solitary exercise, dieting behaviors, and reading and studying.

4. If an adolescent client previously had regular menstrual periods that have been interrupted, it is important to examine both potential medical causes and the possibility of a developing eating disorder.

5. Any evidence of purging calls for further investigation. Sometimes an adolescent will mention an interest in laxative use or self-induced vomiting to a trusted adult, and these are fairly common topics of conversation among female adolescent friends. Purging is a clearly identifiable behavior and is often a good place to start intervening with a young person who is considering or experimenting with unhealthy methods of weight loss. The possible consequences of rotted teeth, a puffy face, and possible heart problems can be convincing to adolescents who are not yet trapped in a severe eating disorder.

Lask and Bryant-Waugh (1993) also suggested several indicators that may help identify adolescents who have problems with eating and may be vulnerable to developing an eating disorder.

1. Determined food avoidances for any reason should at least arouse a clinician's awareness.

2. It is worth paying attention to any weight loss, or even the failure to gain weight, during the period of preadolescent growth, unless there are other physical or emotional problems to explain it.

3. Two or more of the following: (a) preoccupation with body weight; (b) preoccupation with counting calories, grams of fat, or other measures of food intake; (c) distortions in body image; (d) a fear of being fat; (e) self-induced vomiting; (f) excessive exercise; and (g) purging or laxative abuse.

Lask and Bryant-Waugh (1993) tried to develop practical guidelines to help clinicians recognize potential eating disorders, and it is important to look also at troublesome behavior in adolescents that should be differentiated from eating disorders. The simple refusal to eat certain foods is usually understood best as oppositional behavior when it does not involve a preoccupation with body and weight. Second, some disorders among young people involve a widespread refusal to do much of anything, including eating, talking, washing, engaging in social activities, or drinking. This kind of pervasive refusal obviously can indicate a severe disorder, but in this case the refusal to eat is only one part of a widespread breakdown. Third, many young people develop odd kinds of selective eating that can seem strange to adults. If, for example, an adolescent eats only one or two different foods for a period of time but is otherwise at a reasonable weight, this is more likely a general behavioral problem and not an eating disorder. Fourth, depressed adolescents often have a loss of appetite, but this does not involve active food avoidances and fears about body shape.

Differences between Adolescent and Adult Eating Disorders   I present the diagnostic criteria for adult anorexia and bulimia given in DSM-IVTR (American Psychiatric Association, 2000), but then I discuss some important differences in how these disorders appear in adolescent clients.

DSM-IVTR diagnostic criteria for anorexia include (1) a body weight less than 85% of the expected weight or a failure to gain weight, resulting in maintaining a body weight that is less than 85% of the expected weight; (2) fear of gaining weight; (3) body weight disturbance or denial of the seriousness of low body weight; and (4) the absence of three consecutive menstrual cycles in postmenarcheal females.

The criteria for bulimia include (1) repeated episodes of binge eating; (2) recurrent compensatory behaviors, such as vomiting, use of laxatives or diuretics, fasting, or exercise; (3) episodes of binge eating and compensatory behaviors occurring at least twice per week for three months; (4) self-evaluation unduly influenced by body shape and weight; and (5) these disturbances not exclusively occurring in the presence of anorexia; for example, the individual does not have to be underweight.

One reason I included a section on signs of eating disorders was that the strict application of DSM-IVTR diagnostic criteria often results in the failure to identify young people who have significantly disordered eating and who are vulnerable to the development of severe eating disorders. The criterion, for example, of less than 85% of expected weight is difficult to judge in adolescents because of the enormous variability of height and weight gain during normal puberty. A young person can have an eating disorder without showing any weight loss, and the clinician often must make a judgment about whether a client's eating disorder has prevented what should have been a normal weight gain. The criterion of missing three consecutive menstrual cycles is also difficult to apply because menstrual periods are often erratic and unpredictable, especially early in adolescence, and unidentified anorexia may actually have delayed the onset of menstruation. Because the physical consequences of starvation can be more serious during a period of rapid growth, clinicians working with adolescents need to be sensitive to the possibility of subclinical levels of anorexia and bulimia.

Some Special Treatment Issues with Anorexia   Early intervention is important in the treatment of anorexia. There is a huge difference in the hopefulness of prognosis when adolescent eating disorders are treated early in their development compared with treatment started after the disorder has had time to become established. Early intervention carries with it considerable hope of a good outcome, but a chronic eating disorder that lasts into adulthood often results in devastating consequences and is likely to be much more difficult to treat successfully (Lask & Bryant-Waugh, 1993; Wentz, Gillberg, Gillberg, & Rastam, 2000).

The treatment of eating disorders in adolescents requires an interdisciplinary team of clinicians, probably more than with any other disorder. The Society for Adolescent Medicine (Kreipe et al., 1995) has taken a strong position that such a team should consist of physicians, mental health clinicians, nurses, and dietitians. Eating disorders involve so many aspects of a patient's life and are so potentially life-threatening that treatment goals must address several different issues at once, depending on the severity of the disorder and the stage of its development.

Different treatments are needed at different stages of the disorder. By the time most adolescents are formally diagnosed with an eating disorder, they are in such danger of permanent physical damage that medical intervention is absolutely essential to produce weight gain and a return to physical health. Once weight gain has been re-established, or if the disorder is at a less serious stage to start with, the focus of treatment can shift to nutritional counseling and a more psychological focus on problems of distorted body image, self-esteem, and family issues (Lask & Bryant-Waugh, 1993). It might be helpful to think of the early stages of treatment as focused more on control and containment of the acute phases of the problem. In some cases this might involve hospitalization or partial hospitalization (Sanders, 1996) for refeeding, and it probably will involve giving extensive education and information to the adolescent, parents, and other closely involved individuals. Relatively structured behavior modification and family therapy programs can be helpful at this stage. Cognitive behavioral therapy and insight-oriented therapy should be saved until later in the process because they have relatively little effect when a patient is in the grips of starvation (Danziger, Carel, Tyano, & Mimouni, 1989). Robin, Gilroy, and Dennis (1998) say, "There is no evidence for the effectiveness of dynamic or cognitive behavioral individual therapies by themselves in treating children and adolescents with anorexia nervosa, although there is a consensus that both are invaluable components in the middle and later phases of multicomponent intervention" (pp. 441–442).

I have discussed principles of family therapy in chapter 6, but it is worth noting here that the involvement of the family is especially important when treating eating disorders in children and adolescents. Robin, Gilroy, and Dennis (1998) say, "For young adolescents, family therapy where the parents are asked to take charge of their adolescent's eating is more effective in restoring weight than individual therapy in the short run, but as long as the parents are involved in collateral sessions, both treatments work equally well in the long run" (p. 441). Eating disorders can be treated with individual therapy, but eating behavior is so intimately intertwined with family functioning that family therapy should always be considered as a possibility.

Robin and Siegel (1999) list several reasons that family therapy is an essential part of the treatment of eating disorders in adolescents. First, as noted in chapter 1, one primary developmental task during adolescence is separating and individuating from the family. Issues surrounding individuation are often involved in eating disorders, and dealing with them effectively often involves working with the family system. Second, an adolescent with an eating disorder is often confused and unable to think clearly as one result of the semi-starvation. Therefore it is often necessary for the client's family to be persistent, persuasive, and well structured during the refeeding phase of treatment. Third, because the adolescent with an eating disorder often denies even that there is a problem, parents often have to be the ones who make sure that treatment occurs. Finally, it is becoming increasingly difficult to get insurance authorization or support from managed care programs to hospitalize (or even partially hospitalize) patients for the length of time often needed to establish refeeding. Clinicians and parents need to find creative ways to deal with the daunting job of re-establishing a healthy weight for the young patient.

PERSONALITY DISORDERS

In this section I focus on the disorders that are among the most difficult to treat.

How Personality Disorders Differ from Other Problems

Personality disorders are most often described as "characterological" problems. They are long-lasting ways of being a certain way that are inflexible and chronic. Most emotional problems tend to come and go and change, but personality disorders tend to start in childhood and continue throughout life in a way that pervades the person's life. To say that personality disorders are characterological problems implies that they are more part of the person than they are problems that the person has. This difference requires a shift in our thinking as clinicians who treat personality disorders. With other kinds of disorders our goal is more like solving the problem, but personality disorders require us to think in terms of helping a person with a particular character structure live a better life, even though we might not be successful in changing that character structure.

Difficulties Diagnosing Personality Disorders

Because personality disorders differ from other problems primarily because of their chronicity, it is often difficult to draw the line between personality disorders and other kinds of problems. Personality disorders are notoriously difficult to diagnose reliably, and some clinicians seem to use this as a wastebasket category for diagnosing any adolescent who is especially difficult to treat.

Descriptions of Personality Disorders

DSM-IVTR divides personality disorders into three clusters. Cluster A personality disorders are called the odd or eccentric cluster because they include personality patterns that resemble paranoia and schizophrenia. *Paranoid personality disorder* is characterized by a pervasive irrational distrust of others. *Schizoid personality disorder* is characterized by a profound detachment from relationships with other people. *Schizotypal personality disorder* is more severe and includes both the social isolation and beliefs and behaviors that make other people think of the person as odd or bizarre.

Cluster B personality disorders are often described as erratic, emotional, or overly dramatic disorders. *Antisocial personality disorder* is characterized by a pattern of responding to immediate gratification that often leads to such behaviors as cheating friends and family, chronic lying without regard for consequences, and the manipulative exploitation of others without apparent empathy or remorse. *Borderline personality disorder* is characterized by interpersonal tumult, frequent suicidal gestures, and astonishingly erratic swings in emotion. (I discuss antisocial personality disorder and borderline personality disorder in more detail later in this section.) *Histrionic personality disorder* is characterized by overly dramatic behavior. *Narcissistic personality disorder* is characterized by an exaggerated self-importance and a sense of entitlement that comes out of this self-focus.

Cluster C personality disorders are characterized as anxious or fearful. *Avoidant personality disorder* applies to people who are extremely sensitive to the opinions of other people and have extremely low self-esteem that leads them to avoid relationships. *Dependent personality disorder* is characterized by an irrational fear of abandonment and an inability to make decisions and take actions without the approval of others. *Obsessive-compulsive personality disorder* describes people who are consumed by the need for detail and for things to be done "properly."

Many clinicians react to descriptions of various personality disorders with some version of, "They seem like other disorders only worse or more permanent or something." This kind of vague discomfort with understanding personality disorders almost certainly underlies the difficulty in validly diagnosing them. Most of the personality disorders I have discussed resemble other disorders based on painful emotions, especially Cluster A and Cluster C disorders. It is often difficult to decide, for example, when intense mistrustfulness becomes severe enough or "characterological" enough to qualify as a personality disorder. However, two personality disorders stand out as more common and more likely to be difficult for the practicing clinician. They are borderline personality disorder and antisocial personality disorder, and I discuss them in more detail because if you do much clinical practice, you almost certainly will need to deal with them.

Borderline Personality Disorder in Adolescence

The one word that best describes borderline personality disorder is *erratic*. Weiner (1992) discusses six characteristics of the core descriptions of borderline personality disorder: intense emotions, impulsive acts, illusory social adaptation, strained social relationships, brief psychotic episodes, and persistence of the disorder.

The picture of borderline personality disorder can probably best be fleshed out by reading the DSM-IVTR diagnostic criteria for this disorder (American Psychiatric Association, 2000, p. 710):

> A pervasive pattern of instability of interpersonal relationships, self-image, and affects, and marked impulsivity beginning by early adulthood and present in a variety of contexts, as indicated by five (or more) of the following:
> 1. frantic efforts to avoid real or imagined abandonment. Note: Do not include suicidal or self-mutilating behavior covered in Criterion 5.
> 2. a pattern of unstable and intense interpersonal relationships characterized by alternating between extremes of idealization and devaluation
> 3. identity disturbance: markedly and persistently unstable self-image or sense of self
> 4. impulsivity in at least two areas that are potentially self-damaging (e.g., spending, sex, substance abuse, reckless driving, binge eating). Note: Do not include suicidal or self-mutilating behavior covered in Criterion 5.
> 5. recurrent suicidal behavior, gestures, or threats, or self-mutilating behavior
> 6. affective instability due to a marked reactivity of mood (e.g., intense episodic dysphoria, or irritability, or anxiety usually lasting a few hours or only rarely more than a few days)
> 7. chronic feelings of emptiness

8. inappropriate, intense anger or difficulty controlling anger (e.g., frequent displays of temper, constant anger, recurrent physical fights)
9. transient, stress-related paranoid ideation or severe disassociative symptoms

Special Treatment Issues   In previous chapters I quoted several researchers who noted that psychotherapy with adolescent clients is especially difficult. Many clinicians would say that whether you have adult clients or adolescent clients, the most demanding and difficult therapy is the treatment of personality disorders, especially borderline personality disorder. Shay (1987) titled one of his articles "The Wish to Do Psychotherapy with Borderline Adolescents— And Other Common Errors." He says, "Most clinicians would agree that psychotherapy with adolescents, especially borderline adolescents, is an extremely difficult undertaking" (p. 718). Actually, he didn't mean that it was necessarily an error to treat adolescents with borderline personality disorder but that such treatment is difficult partly because the things we know most to do in therapy are not particularly effective with these clients. Many clinicians approach psychotherapy with their adolescent clients by offering interpretations and intellectual insights and by acting "shrinky," as many personality-disordered adolescents describe their previous therapists.

Treating adolescents with borderline personality disorder requires enormous patience, resilience, and the wise application of techniques that will be quite different from your experience in treating other kinds of problems. I do not mean any of this to be discouraging or to imply that borderline personality cannot or should not be treated; the opposite is the truth. However, you also need to know the truth that in the real world many clinicians are reluctant to treat people with borderline personality disorder, because the process can be so demanding, exhausting, and frustrating. Of course, there are also clinicians who say the same thing about treating any adolescents. Some clinicians are wonderfully effective with adolescents, and some do very well treating borderline personality disorder. You will need to discover for yourself if you are suited to it.

Another treatment issue is *splitting.* Fall and Craig (1998) say that "the nature of the disorder precludes the effective use of the counseling relationship to aid in the treatment" (p. 322). This characteristic of borderline personality disorder is called splitting, in which the person adopts an all-or-none dichotomous view of the world. Unpredictably, your client may express intense respect and caring for you at one point and then seem to turn on you without warning and tell you and anyone else who will listen how horrible you are. Sometimes this will clearly be in response to something the clinician has done that the client perceives as not sufficiently attentive or as insensitive or unacceptable for some other reason. Sometimes, however, there will be no obvious reason for the sudden intense change.

The most obvious difference between treating borderline personality disorders and other problems is the absolute necessity for the clinician to consistently set, maintain, and enforce reasonable limits on the therapy relationship and on what the client can do within the therapy relationship. You will still need to be both firm and reassuring, but your emphasis will dramatically shift toward firmness compared with your treating other kinds of problems. Manipulative suicide attempts are not uncommon with borderline personality disorder, for example, and you will need to have a way to deal with these that does not allow you to be manipulated but also responsibly protects your client from harm. You might, for example, arrange for the police always to deal with such attempts rather than becoming involved in them yourself. It will be especially important that these and other manipulative attempts do not work by getting you to violate your limits with special favors or new arrangements. You might have a client who repeatedly phones you at 2 A.M., frantic and desperate to talk. Sometimes, of course, this might reflect an emergency that requires intervention. However, your response to it must not encourage such behavior. You might say, for example, "I cannot and will not talk at this time. I do hear that you need to talk, but you may not call me in the middle of the night to talk. If you need to go to the hospital, call 911. Otherwise, I would be willing to see you in my office tomorrow." (I am assuming here that making an appointment for tomorrow would not be yielding to manipulation.) Many clinicians will find it difficult to hold the line this firmly without feeling harsh and untherapeutic. However, if you cannot hold firm and reasonable limits with your clients, you will be doing them damage by reinforcing their destructive behavior, and you will eventually find it impossible to treat borderline personality disorder because you will burn out.

The focus of treatment with borderline personality disorder is not on self-exploration and insight. It is on reality-based problem solving about coping skills and it involves significantly more confrontation from the clinician (Fall & Craig, 1998; Weiner, 1992). Linehan (1993) described an approach, called dialectical behavior therapy

(DBT), for borderline personality disorder that is consistent with the principles I have been discussing. DBT was originally developed to reduce suicidal gestures, but it has been broadened to include methods to retain the client in treatment and to improve interpersonal behaviors. DBT includes individual therapy, group skills training time, weekly case consultations with other professionals involved with the client, and telephone consultations between the clinician and the client between individual sessions. The focus of treatment is on concrete problem solving, but Linehan is clear that the work must be founded on the clinician's clear belief in the client's ability to change. The clinician must find a way to instill that belief in the client if treatment is to be effective. This is done primarily through the validation of the client by focusing on the positive aspects of the client's current problem solving that is working and behaviors and emotions that are effective. By working to identify these positive aspects of the client and to identify stressors in the client's life, much of the blame and judgment are taken out of the process without losing the highly structured problem-oriented approach.

Antisocial Personality Disorder in Adolescence

Antisocial personality disorder is the correct and current term for what used to be called psychopathy or sociopathy. This disorder is marked by an apparent lack of normal feelings of conscience, empathy for others, and trustworthiness. The person's behavior seems largely governed by immediate gratification, with little or no concern for long-term consequences to self or others. It fits the general description of personality disorders, in that it is "an enduring pattern of inner experience and behavior that deviates markedly from the expectations of the individual's culture" (American Psychiatric Association, 2000, p. 686), but this disorder seems markedly different from the other personality disorders in one overwhelmingly important way. Most of the other personality disorders seem to be marked by attempts to ward off painful emotions such as anxiety, fear of abandonment, and deep insecurities. In other words, they seem to be based on too much painful emotion that has molded the person's core character and against which the person has developed defenses. Antisocial personality disorder seems more understandable as the opposite; it seems as though the person experiences too little emotion. It may seem odd to say so, but we do need some level of anxiety, guilt, and sensitivity to the pain of others in order to live with other people in society.

All of this has enormous implications for the treatment of anti-social personality disorder. To say it simplistically, most of our treatments are designed to reduce and control painful emotions. If the problem stems from too little emotion in the first place, some of the things that clinicians normally do might well make an antisocial personality disorder problem worse. This is a sobering thought. Among adolescents it is more common to find a diagnosis of conduct disorder, but this label "is so broad a diagnostic category, encompassing so many different kinds of behaviors, that it requires more sophistication to avoid the diagnosis than make it" (Lewis, 1997, p. 441).

Not All Antisocial Behavior Is Antisocial Personality Disorder or Conduct Disorder   Many, if not most, of the adolescent clients whom you treat will do things that most people would call antisocial, but few of them will fit the description or the dynamics of antisocial personality disorder or conduct disorder. Some antisocial behavior occurs because it is socialized; most other people in the adolescent's environment behave in the same way, and the antisocial behavior is strongly reinforced in the adolescent's subculture or personal environment. In many ways this kind of antisocial behavior is completely normal in the person's environment. You and I would probably do the same things if we had grown up the same way. In other cases antisocial behavior can be a reaction to anxiety, insecurity, depression, or other painful emotions. It can be a bid for attention or serve to distract the person from other problems. In other words, much—probably most—of the antisocial behavior you see in the adolescents you treat is not the result of antisocial personality disorder.

Clearly, you are faced with a difficult dilemma that requires you to be especially sensitive in your assessment of your clients' problems. In most cases you will be doing your clients a disservice by treating them as though they had antisocial personality disorder, but relationship-based and anxiety-reducing treatment methods could make the problem worse if the client does have antisocial personality disorder or a conduct disorder based on a tendency to respond primarily to immediate gratification.

Special Treatment Considerations   Attempts to treat antisocial personality disorder with relationship-based therapy are notoriously unsuccessful (Lewis, 1997; Kazdin, 1987). Lewis (1997) says, "To date, no specific treatment has proved effective for adolescents with conduct disorder despite the numerous approaches that have been taken" (p. 451). Kazdin (1987) concluded that "no particular approach has been shown to ameliorate antisocial behavior" (p. 74). These problems are probably best dealt with through highly structured and controlled programs that stress problem solving and immediate rewards for prosocial behavior, combined with strict limits and immediate consequences for antisocial behavior.

SCHIZOPHRENIA IN ADOLESCENTS

My goal in this section is not to equip you to diagnose schizophrenia, but it is important that you be able to recognize the major characteristics of schizophrenia in the young people with whom you are working. An understanding of the symptoms and some of the causes of schizophrenia will help you to understand some of the differences in treating schizophrenia and other kinds of disorders.

Common Symptoms

Premorbid Symptoms   Most adolescents who are eventually diagnosed with schizophrenia will have shown prior behaviors that made people think of them as "odd" children. They frequently will have had difficulties with social relationships, been withdrawn, done poorly in school, and demonstrated unusual kinds of thinking.

Positive Symptoms   Symptoms of schizophrenia can be roughly divided into two categories: negative symptoms and positive symptoms. Negative symptoms refer to deficits in behavior compared to what we would expect from a normal person. They include flat affect, social withdrawal, alogia, and avolition. I discuss these later in this section. Positive symptoms refer to the unusual and observable behaviors that appear during active episodes of schizophrenia. Positive symptoms are more obvious and therefore easier to describe than negative symptoms. Examples of positive symptoms are hallucinations, delusions, thought disorder, and bizarre behavior. I discuss each of these in the following paragraphs.

Hallucinations are perceptions that the person experiences as real things in the external environment without the presence of an actual external stimulus. Hallucinations can involve any of the five senses: sounds (auditory hallucinations), images (visual hallucinations), physical sensations (tactile hallucinations), tastes (gustatory hallucinations), or odors (olfactory hallucinations). In general, hallucinations are the most common symptom of schizophrenia, and auditory hallucinations are more common than any other kind. The patient often hears voices saying specific things, hears frightening sounds such as footsteps coming down the hall, or hears sounds that are clear but difficult to describe. Visual hallucinations can include seeing people and objects that are not actually present, but these are unusual enough to warrant checking for neurological difficulties other than schizophrenia. Tactile hallucinations might include the clear sensation of bugs crawling on a person's skin or more general sensations such as a feeling of pressure. The perceptions of tastes and odors are even more rare, but they do occur.

Two kinds of hallucinations that often occur in people with no psychiatric illness are hypnogogic hallucinations, which can occur when a person is falling asleep, or hypnopompic hallucinations, which can occur as the person is waking up. These hallucinations can be vivid and seem quite real and are often especially frightening to young people who are sometimes relieved to learn that they can be quite normal.

Delusions are strongly held beliefs that have no foundation in reality and are not believed by other members of the person's culture. Delusions are a common characteristic of schizophrenia among adult patients, but they are less frequently seen in adolescents. Delusions of persecution and delusions regarding the body seem to be the most frequent ones associated with schizophrenia. A person might believe, for example, that the police have secretly implanted a tracking device under his or her skin and are gathering evidence against the person. There are, of course, thousands of potential delusions that a person might hold, but their defining characteristic is that they contradict all reasonable evidence and they will not yield to rational persuasion. The person is truly and absolutely convinced of their truth.

One of the clearest indicators of schizophrenia is thought disorder, which is often referred to as cognitive slippage. It is almost as though the person's verbal processes are short-circuiting. Sometimes this results in loose associations in which the person might say something such as, "People say you can be whatever you want to be, but bees are insects." The person seems to have trouble inhibiting odd associations from one word to another. Cognitive slippage can also appear as illogical speech, such as, "I don't want dinner because people don't care about the rain." Finally, thought disorder can appear as impoverished speech patterns in which the person seems unable to think of appropriate words. For example, the person might say, "I want a . . . sort of one of . . . to go on with . . . something."

Individuals with schizophrenia may remain immobilized for long periods in odd positions. This immobility is called catatonia. More likely, however, patients with schizophrenia will perform bizarre behaviors that draw attention to them because they so blatantly violate normal social conventions. These can range from relatively innocuous acts, such as picking at the air for things that aren't there, to behavior that will almost inevitably get the person in legal difficulty, such as disrobing in a restaurant or acting in frightening, impulsive ways in response to their delusions and hallucinations.

Negative Symptoms   As I noted, negative symptoms refer to deficits in behavior compared to what we would expect from a normal person. Typical negative symptoms are flat affect, social withdrawal, alogia, and avolition.

An adolescent with schizophrenia often appears profoundly bland emotionally. Affect is frequently described as blunted or flat because the person's speech, expressions, and behaviors seem devoid of emotion. Although this lack of normal response to social cues is most typical, the person may swing the opposite direction and display inappropriate emotion by laughing for no apparent reason or smiling and giggling in sad situations.

A lack of friendships and other social relationships is characteristic of schizophrenia, and the person frequently loses friendships that existed before the appearance of schizophrenia. This asocial way of being is partly the result of other people having difficulty dealing with the person's oddness, but it is probably caused more by characteristics of the person with schizophrenia. There seems to be a lack of motivation and ability to start new relationships. It seems likely that the process of forming relationships feels daunting and frightening to the person with schizophrenia.

When I described thought disorder earlier, I mentioned an inability to find words to express a particular thought. This inability is one example of alogia, a general impoverishment of thought processes. A person with schizophrenia generally tends to say less in general and seems to be struggling to think while speaking. There may be uncomfortably long pauses and frequent interruptions in the person's speech.

A general lack of motivation (avolition) often occurs with schizophrenia, and the person may neglect personal hygiene and may fail to follow through on activities.

Special Treatment Issues

Schizophrenia among adolescents is difficult to treat, but about 25% of adolescents who have been hospitalized for schizophrenia recover; another 25% show significant improvement but do not have a full recovery. Thus the prognosis for schizophrenia among hospitalized adolescents is not as optimistic as it is among adults hospitalized for schizophrenia; only approximately 25% of adult patients do not show a full or partial recovery. Although these statistics can be seen as discouraging, they also suggest significant hope for the value of treatment of schizophrenia in adolescence.

Medical Intervention   There is little doubt that genetic and biochemical factors are involved with schizophrenia, and any treatment program for an adolescent with schizophrenia should involve medical consultation and, in most cases, the use of antipsychotic drugs. These medications are especially helpful with adolescents in the acute stages of schizophrenia and especially when positive symptoms are strong. Schizophrenia characterized primarily by negative symptoms or by symptoms that have lasted so long that they could be called chronic does not respond as well to medications. Antipsychotic medications are most effective at reducing agitation and anxiety, and they have a calming effect that includes the reduction of cognitive slippage. The increased ability to think logically often makes the adolescent more accessible to psychotherapy (Weiner, 1992).

Most medical practitioners urge that antipsychotic medications be used conservatively, especially with young patients. The medications have a number of distressing side effects, and adolescents frequently resist them because of these side effects. Medications should always be considered a likely part of treatment, but they should be regarded as an adjunct to support and facilitate other kinds of treatment using multiple modalities. Drugs often provide a context within which a young person can learn new social skills, increase personal understanding, and be empowered by taking responsibility for more of his or her own treatment and life.

Psychological Treatment   The treatment of an adolescent with schizophrenia must be multifaceted. In addition to the judicious use of medications, treatment should include group experiences that both teach new social skills and increase comfort in social situations (Thienemann & Shaw, 1996), practical and highly structured experiences that teach practical skills in living, and, ideally, some kind of individual psychotherapy (Campbell et al., 1997).

Weiner (1992) says that adolescent schizophrenia includes two features that are especially appropriate for psychotherapy: difficulties with interpersonal relationships and distortions of reality. An understanding of these two characteristics leads to his description of the two primary tasks a therapist undertakes in treating an adolescent with schizophrenia. The first step is relationship building, and the second step is reality testing.

Establishing a therapeutic relationship with a teenager who has schizophrenia is a delicate business. The client is usually withdrawn from relationships in general and has poor interpersonal skills. It is probably not an exaggeration to say that most of the young people are terrified of connecting with another person. You will, of course, use all the skills we have discussed in this book to help your client know you as understanding, accepting, and honest. However, communicating these qualities requires a gentle attunement that respects the client's deep fear of relating. It requires sensitivity to the impact of almost everything the therapist does and says. Just as important as this sensitivity is, you will need not to be weak and permissive in the face of disruptive or destructive words and actions. It is often said that the ideal parent is firm and loving, and some version of these qualities, perhaps understanding and accepting combined with dependable, gentle firmness, probably describes the ideal therapist for a young person with schizophrenia.

A great gift that a clinician can give to an adolescent with schizophrenia is to make it easy simply to talk. Adolescents with schizophrenia typically are withdrawn from others and often refuse to say much of anything to anybody. It is difficult for others to imagine the intensity of fear and pain that comes from not being in control of one's own rational thinking, but it seems likely that this fear of chaotic confusion is part of what motivates a person with schizophrenia to avoid social interactions. Often, the sensitive clinician can pick up on topics that the client is able to think about and explain clearly. These topics might well be something fairly simple that interests the client, such as sewing or fishing or a particular memory about which the client is clear. The clinician can listen for and perhaps paraphrase the sensible part of what the client has said. By showing interest in this topic, the clinician is doing something very important: rewarding the client for rational talking. This has an important beneficial effect because it strengthens both rational thinking and talking to other people. To an outside observer these interactions might not look like therapy or be the kind of "working on issues" that we often associate with the therapy process, but they can significantly improve the client's level of comfort and overt behaviors. In chapter 3 I mentioned one young man with schizophrenia who was fascinated by and knowledgeable about the stock market. We spent hours talking about the stock market, and he explained to me (often more than once, in response to my painfully limited understanding of the stock market) much about the financial world. This experience clearly made it more comfortable for him to talk with people in general.

Besides relationship building, Weiner (1992) noted the need for reality testing in treating schizophrenic adolescents. He said that "therapists need to provide schizophrenic adolescents with continual and direct corrections of their distorted perceptions" (p. 92). Of course, this is not accomplished with accusatory confrontations or dismissing the distorted perceptions. Nor is it accomplished with a permissive acceptance of the perceptions as valid and real. The therapist expresses understanding of the reality of the experience for the client and in the same breath communicates that most people, including the therapist, perceive things differently.

Structured and Cognitive Rather Than Emotionally Arousing   For the practicing clinician the most important and useful piece of information about treating adolescents with schizophrenia is to understand that emotionally arousing interactions often make things worse for the client. It is still vitally important that your client feel understood and accepted, but there are many ways to make this happen. In earlier chapters I spent a lot of time talking about how the clinician listens for what the adolescent has implied, especially the experiential and emotional parts of the message. Relating helpfully to a person with schizophrenia also involves responding to what he or she has implied, but it is better to respond in structured and cognitive ways to the implied meaning. Schizophrenia often makes the person vulnerable to frightening emotions that seem chaotic, unstructured, and uncontrollable. Arousing implied feelings can easily overwhelm the person's resources and cause him or her enough pain and turmoil to force further withdrawal and exacerbation of symptoms.

Roth and Fonagy (1996) note that "whereas supportive individual therapy may be helpful for schizophrenic patients, expressive psychotherapy is unlikely to be of value" (p. 195). My experience and the writings of, for example, Fromm-Reichmann (1950) and Sullivan (1962)—both rare therapists with reputations for success treating schizophrenia—suggest that reality-based structuring and focusing are needed rather than evocative arousal and facing of internal conflicts. In a sense, defenses need to be strengthened rather than faced and gotten through.

It might be useful to contrast possible ways to respond to similar verbalizations by two different clients. If a client with an anxiety problem said, "I don't know how to act when I enter a room full of people I don't know," the clinician might respond, "I get a sense that you feel awkward and afraid of what's going to happen, and that confuses you." This response clearly shows that the clinician understood the content of the client's comment and was able to go beyond the words to understand the implied feelings in it. The clinician's response helps the client to face and to deal with the feelings and facilitates the process of problem solving. However, if a young person with schizophrenia said, "I don't know how to act when I enter a room full of people I don't know," a response that focuses on and arouses implicit emotions could easily be so stimulating as to overwhelm the client, who is already having difficulty making sense out of things. You could make this client feel understood and help give structure to the thought by saying, for example, "So you would like to figure out what to do in that situation. We could talk about some things you might do." The clinician's focus here is far more on concrete, more easily articulated behaviors.

WHAT IT ALL BOILS DOWN TO

We have covered a lot of ground together. We have discussed techniques, adolescent psychology, behavioral principles, special circumstances, and different formats for treatment. But we have to end by returning to the essence of what makes all of these tools worth even thinking about. Nothing works unless you can connect with your adolescent client. If you can connect, many things will work. How can you connect? First, your fundamental beliefs about people, especially adolescent people, will drive and inform everything you do. If you do not start from a position of trusting, it will not matter what else you learn. If you do start from a position of trust, you demonstrate that you believe in your clients and you earn their trust. As they begin to trust you and your wish to know them as they are, they will work with you to find ways to go where they need to go.

Recommended Reading

Hsu, L. K. G. (1990). *Eating disorders.* New York: Guilford Press.

Kazdin, A. E. (1987). *Conduct disorders in childhood and adolescence* (v. 9). Newbury Park, CA: Sage.

Lask, B., & Bryant-Waugh, R. (Eds.). (1993). *Childhood onset anorexia and related eating disorders.* Hillsdale, NJ: Lawrence Erlbaum Associates.

Linehan, M. M. (1993). *Cognitive behavioral treatment of personality disorders.* New York: Guilford Press.

Steiner, H. (Ed.). (1996). *Treating adolescents.* San Francisco: Jossey-Bass.

Weiner, I. B. (1992). *Psychological disturbance in adolescence* (2d ed.). New York: Wiley.

BIBLIOGRAPHY

American Psychiatric Association. (2000). *Diagnostic and statistical manual of mental disorders: Text revision* (4th ed.). Washington, DC: American Psychiatric Association.

Angus, L. E., & Rennie, D. L. (1989). Envisioning the representational world: The client's experience of metaphoric expression in psychotherapy. *Psychotherapy, 26,* 372–379.

Azima, F. J. (1989). Confrontation, empathy, and interpretation issues in adolescent group psychotherapy. In F. J. Azima and L. H. Richmond (Eds.), *Adolescent group psychotherapy* (pp. 3–20). American Group Psychotherapy Association Monograph 4. Madison, WI: International Universities Press.

———, & Richmond, L. H. (Eds.). (1989). *Adolescent group psychotherapy.* American Group Psychotherapy Association Monograph 4. Madison, WI: International Universities Press.

Bachelor, A. (1988). How clients perceive therapist empathy: A content analysis of "received" empathy. *Psychotherapy, 25,* 227–240.

Beavers, W. R., & Hampson, R. B. (1990). *Successful families: Assessment and intervention.* New York: Norton.

Bell, J. E. (1963). A theoretical position for family group therapy. *Family Process, 2,* 1–14.

Bleiberg, E. (1994, Spring). Borderline disorders in children and adolescents: The concept, the diagnosis, and the controversies. *Bulletin of the Menninger Clinic, 58*(2), 169–197.

Blos, P. (1962). *On adolescence: A psychoanalytic interpretation.* New York: Free Press of Glencoe.

Bohart, A. C. (1993). Experiencing: The basis of psychotherapy. *Journal of Psychotherapy Integration, 3,* 51–67.

———, & Tallman, K. (1999). *How clients make therapy work.* Washington, DC: American Psychological Association.

Brodsky, S. L., & Lichtenstein, B. (1999). Don't ask questions: A psychotherapeutic strategy for treatment of involuntary clients. *American Journal of Psychotherapy, 53,* 215–221.

Burgum, M. (1942). The father gets worse: A child guidance problem. *American Journal of Orthopsychiatry, 12,* 474–486.

Burns, D. D., & Auerbach, A. (1996). Therapeutic empathy in cognitive-behavioral therapy. In P. M. Salkovskis (Ed.), *Frontiers of cognitive therapy* (pp. 135–164). New York: Guilford Press.

———, & Nolen-Hoeksema, S. (1991). Coping styles, homework compliance, and the effectiveness of cognitive behavioral therapy. *Journal of Consulting and Clinical Psychology, 59,* 305–311.

Campbell, M., Armenteros, J. L., Spencer, E. K., Kowalik, S. C., & Erlenmeyer-Kimling, L. (1997). Schizophrenia and psychotic disorders. In J. M. Weiner (Ed.), *Textbook of child and adolescent psychiatry* (2d ed.) (pp. 303–332). Washington, DC: American Psychiatric Press.

Carkhuff, R. R., & Berenson, B. G. (1977). *Beyond counseling and therapy* (2d ed.). New York: Holt, Rinehart & Winston.

Cirillo, L., & Crider, C. (1995). Distinctive therapeutic uses of metaphor. *Psychotherapy, 32,* 511–519.

Colapinto, J. (1991). Structural family therapy. In A. S. Gurman and S. Knistern (Eds.), *Handbook of family therapy* (pp. 417–443). New York: Brunner/Mazel.

Danziger, Y., Carcl, C. A., Tyano, S., & Mimouni, M. (1989). Is psychotherapy mandatory during the acute refeeding in the treatment of anorexia nervosa? *Journal of Adolescent Health Care, 10,* 328–331.

Eaton, T. T., Abeles, N., & Gutfreund, M. J. (1988). Therapeutic alliance and outcome: Impact of treatment length and pretreatment symptomatology. *Psychotherapy, 25,* 536–542.

Ellis, A. (1994). *Reason and emotion in psychotherapy* (rev. ed.). New York: Carol.

Erikson, E. H. (1956). The problem of ego identity. *Journal of the American Psychoanalytic Association, 4,* 56–121.

Fall, K. A., & Craig, S. E. (1998). Borderline personality in adolescence: An overview for counselors. *Journal of Mental Health Counseling, 20,* 315–332.

Freud, A. (1936/1946). *The ego and the mechanisms of defense.* New York: International Universities Press.

———. (1969). Adolescence as a developmental disturbance. In S. Lebovici & G. Caplan (Eds.), *Adolescence: Psychological perspectives* (pp. 5–10). New York: Basic Books.

Fromm-Reichmann, F. (1950). *Principles of intensive psychotherapy.* Chicago: Phoenix Books, University of Chicago Press.

Garfield, S. L. (1986). Problems in diagnostic classification. In T. Millon and G. L. Klerman (Eds.), *Contemporary directions in psychopathology* (pp. 99–114). New York: Guilford Press.

Guldner, C. A. (1990). Family therapy with adolescents. *Journal of Group Psychotherapy, Psychodrama & Sociometry, 43,* 142–153.

Gurman, A. S. (1977). The patient's perceptions of the therapeutic relationship. In A. S. Gurman & A. M. Razin (Eds.), *Effective psychotherapy: A handbook of research* (pp. 503–543). Oxford: Pergamon Press.

Hall, G. S. (1904). *Adolescence: Its psychology and its relations to physiology, anthropology, sociology, sex, crime, religion, and education* (2 vols.). New York: D. Appleton.

Havas, E., & Bonnar, D. (1999). Therapy with adolescents and families: The limits of parenting. *American Journal of Family Therapy, 27,* 121–135.

Hibbs, E. D., & Jensen, P. S. (1996). *Psychosocial treatments for child and adolescent disorders.* Washington, DC: American Psychological Association.

Horvath, A. O., & Luborsky, L. (1993). The role of the therapeutic alliance in psychotherapy. *Journal of Consulting and Clinical Psychology, 61,* 561–573.

Hsu, L. K. G. (1990). *Eating disorders.* New York: Guilford Press.

Kahn, B. B. (1999). Art therapy with adolescents: Making it work for school counselors. *Professional School Counseling, 2,* 291–299.

Katz, P. (1990). The first few minutes: The engagement of the difficult adolescent. In S. C. Feinstein (Ed.), *Adolescent psychiatry: Developmental and clinical studies* (v. 17, pp. 69–81). Chicago: University of Chicago Press.

———. (1998). Establishing the therapeutic alliance. In A. H. Esman (Ed.), *Adolescent psychiatry: Developmental and clinical studies* (v. 23, pp. 89–105). Hillsdale, NJ: Analytic Press.

Kazdin, A. E. (1987). *Conduct disorders in childhood and adolescence* (v. 9). Newbury Park, CA: Sage.

Kreipe, R. E., Golden, N. G., Katzman, D. K., Fisher, M., Rees, J., Tonkin, R. S., et al. (1995). Eating disorders in adolescents: A position paper of the Society for Adolescent Medicine. *Journal of Adolescent Health, 16,* 476–480.

L'Abate, L., and Bagarozzi, D. A. (1993). *Sourcebook of marriage and family evaluation.* New York: Brunner/Mazel.

Lambert, M. J., Bergin, A. E., & Collins, J. L. (1977). Therapist-induced deterioration in psychotherapy. In A. S. Gurman & A. M. Razin (Eds.),

Effective psychotherapy: A handbook of research (pp. 452–481). Oxford: Pergamon Press.

Lask, B., & Bryant-Waugh, R. (Eds.). (1993). *Childhood onset anorexia and related eating disorders.* Hillsdale, NJ: Lawrence Erlbaum Associates.

Lewinsohn, P. M., & Clarke, G. N. (1999). Psychosocial treatments for adolescent depression. *Clinical Psychology Review,* 19, 329–342.

Lewis, D. O. (1997). Conduct and antisocial disorders in adolescence. In J. M. Weiner (Ed.), *Textbook of child and adolescent psychiatry* (2d ed.) (pp. 441–458). Washington, DC: American Psychiatric Press.

Liddle, H. A. (1995). Conceptual and clinical dimensions of a multidimensional, multisystems engagement strategy in family-based adolescent treatment. *Psychotherapy,* 32, 39–58.

Linehan, M. M. (1993). *Cognitive-behavioral treatment of personality disorders.* New York: Guilford Press.

Lock, J. (1996). Depression, In H. Steiner (Ed.), *Treating adolescents* (pp. 153–186). San Francisco: Jossey-Bass.

Maccoby, E. E., & Martin, J. A. (1983). Socialization in the context of the family: Parent-child interaction. In P. H. Mussen (Ed.), *Handbook of child psychology* (v. 4, pp. 1–101). New York: Wiley.

Martin, D. G. (1969). Consistency of self-descriptions under different role sets among neurotic and normal adolescents and adults. *Journal of Abnormal Psychology,* 74, 173–176.

———. (2000). *Counseling and therapy skills* (2d ed.). Prospect Heights, IL: Waveland Press.

Martin, G., & Pear, J. (1998). *Behavior modification: What it is and how to do it* (6th ed.). Englewood Cliffs, NJ: Prentice Hall.

Meeks, J. E. (1997). Psychotherapy of the adolescent. In L. T. Flaherty and R. M. Sarles, *Handbook of child and adolescent psychiatry* (v. 3, pp. 381–394). New York: Wiley.

Meyer, J. H., & Zegans, L. W. (1975). Adolescents perceive their psychotherapy. *Psychiatry,* 38, 11–22.

Micucci, J. A. (1998). *The adolescent in family therapy.* New York: Guilford Press.

Miller, I. W., Kabacoff, R. I., Epstein, N. B., Bishop, D. S., Keitner, G. I., Baldwon, L. M., et al. (1994). The development of a clinical rating scale of the McMaster Model of Family Functioning. *Family Process,* 33, 53–69.

Minuchin, S. (1974). *Families and family therapy.* Cambridge: Harvard University Press.

Mohr, D. C. (1995). Negative outcome in psychotherapy: A critical review. *Clinical Psychology: Science and Practice,* 2, 1–27.

Morris, R. J., & Nicholson, J. (1993). The therapeutic relationship in child and adolescent psychotherapy: Research issues and trends. In T. R. Kratochwill & R. J. Morris (Eds.), *Handbook of psychotherapy with chil-*

dren and adolescents (pp. 405–425). Needham Heights, MA: Allyn and Bacon.

Najavits, L. M., & Strupp, H. H. (1994). Differences in the effectiveness of psychodynamic therapists: A process-outcome study. *Psychotherapy,* 31, 114–123.

Nichols, W. C. (1999). Family systems therapy. In S. W. Russ & T. H. Ollendick (Eds.), *Handbook of psychotherapies with children and families* (pp. 137–151). New York: Plenum Press.

Offer, D., Ostrov, E., & Howard, K. I. (1981). The mental health professional's concept of the normal adolescent. *Archives of General Psychiatry,* 38, 149–152.

———, & Sabshin, M. (1984). Adolescence: Empirical perspectives. In D. Offer & M. Sabshin (Eds.), *Normality and the life cycle* (pp. 76–107). New York: Basic Books.

Ornston, P. S., Cicchetti, D., Levine, J., & Fierman, L. B. (1968). Some parameters of verbal behavior that reliably differentiate novice from experienced psychotherapists. *Journal of Abnormal Psychology,* 73, 240–244.

Petersen, A. C. (1988). Adolescent development. *Annual Review of Psychology,* 39, 583–607.

Pitta, P. (1995). Adolescent-centered family integrated philosophy and treatment. *Psychotherapy,* 32, 99–107.

Powers, S. I., Hauser, S. T., & Kilner, L. A. (1989). Adolescent mental health. *American Psychologist,* 44, 200–208.

Reinecke, M. A. (1993). Outpatient treatment of mild psychopathology. In P. H. Tolan & B. J. Cohler (Eds.), *Handbook of clinical research and practice with adolescents* (pp. 387–410). New York: Wiley.

Robin, A. L., Gilroy, M., & Dennis, A. B. (1998). Treatment of eating disorders in children and adolescents. *Clinical Psychology Review,* 18, 421–446.

———, & Siegel, P. T. (1999). Family therapy with eating-disordered adolescents. In S. W. Russ & T. H. Ollendick (Eds.), *Handbook of psychotherapies with children and families* (pp. 301–325). New York: Plenum Press.

Rogers, C. R. (1975). Empathic: An unappreciated way of being. *Counseling Psychologist,* 5, 2–10.

———. (1980). Client-centered psychotherapy. In H. I. Kaplan, B. J. Sadock, & A. M. Freedman (Eds.), *Comprehensive textbook of psychiatry* (v. 3, pp. 2153–2186). Baltimore: Williams & Wilkins.

Roth, A., & Fonagy, P. (1996). *What works for whom? A critical review of psychotherapy research.* New York: Guilford Press.

Sanders, M. J. (1996). Eating disorders. In H. Steiner (Ed.), *Treating adolescents* (pp. 223–260). San Francisco: Jossey-Bass.

Schniering, C. A., Hudson, J. L., & Rapee, R. M. (2000). Issues in the diagnosis and assessment of anxiety disorders in children and adolescents. *Clinical Psychology Review, 20,* 453–478.

Schubert, J. (1977). *The therapeutic interview.* Unpublished manuscript, University of Regina, Regina, Canada.

Shambaugh, P. W. (1996). Developmental models of adolescent groups. In P. Kymissis & D. A. Halperin (Eds.), *Group therapy with children and adolescents* (pp. 55–75). Washington, DC: American Psychiatric Press.

Shay, J. J. (1987). The wish to do psychotherapy with borderline adolescents—and other common errors. *Psychotherapy, 24,* 712–719.

Sholevar, G. P. (1997). Family therapy. In J. M. Wiener (Ed.), *Textbook of child and adolescent psychiatry* (2d ed.) (pp. 103–115). Washington, DC: American Psychiatric Press.

Smith, D., & Dumont, F. (1995). A cautionary study: Unwarranted interpretations of the Draw-a-Person Test. *Professional Psychology, 26,* 298–303.

Sommers-Flanagan, J., & Sommers-Flanagan, R. (1995). Psychotherapeutic techniques with treatment-resistant adolescents. *Psychotherapy, 32,* 131–140.

———. (1997). *Tough kids, cool counseling.* Alexandria, VA: American Counseling Association.

Soo, E. S. (1996). Supervision. In P. Kymissis & D. A. Halperin (Eds.), *Group therapy with children and adolescents* (pp. 111–132). Washington, DC: American Psychiatric Press.

Spiegel, S. (1996). *An interpersonal approach to child and adolescent psychotherapy.* Northvale, NJ: Jason Aronson.

Spiegler, M. D., & Guevremont, D. C. (1998). *Contemporary behavior therapy* (3d ed.). Pacific Grove, CA: Brooks/Cole.

Stein, M. D., & Kymissis, P. (1989). Adolescent inpatient group psychotherapy. In F. J. Azima & L. H. Richmond (Eds.), *Adolescent group psychotherapy* (pp. 69–83). American Group Psychotherapy Association Monograph 4. Madison, WI: International Universities Press.

Strome, S. S., & Loutsch, E. M. (1996). A structured, educative form of adolescent psychotherapy. In P. Kymissis, & D. A. Halperin (Eds.), *Group therapy with children and adolescents* (pp. 175–187). Washington, DC: American Psychiatric Press.

Sullivan, H. S. (1962). *Schizophrenia as a human process.* New York: Norton.

Swift, W. J. (1993). Brief psychotherapy with adolescents: Individual and family approaches. *American Journal of Psychotherapy, 47,* 373–387.

Thienemann, M., & Shaw, R. J. (1996). Schizophrenia and psychotic disorders. In H. Steiner (Ed.), *Treating adolescents* (pp. 309–344). San Francisco: Jossey-Bass.

Toth, J. P., & Reingold, E. M. (1996). Beyond perception: Conceptual contributions to unconscious influences of memory. In G. Underwood (Ed.), *Implicit cognition* (pp. 41–84). Oxford: Oxford University Press.

Turner, J. T., Batik, M., Palmer, L. J., Forbes, D, & McDermott, B. M. (2000). Detection and importance of laxative use in adolescents with anorexia nervosa. *Journal of the American Academy of Child and Adolescent Psychiatry*, 39, 378–385.

Vanaerschot, G. (1997). Empathic resonance as a source of experience-enhancing interventions. In A. C. Bohart & L. S. Greenberg, *Empathy reconsidered* (pp. 141–165). Washington, DC: American Psychological Association.

Vraniak, D., & Pickett, S. (1993). Improving interventions with American ethnic minority children: Recurrent and recalcitrant challenges. In T. Kratochwill & R. Morris (Eds.), *Handbook of psychotherapy with children and adolescents* (pp. 502–540). Boston: Allyn & Bacon.

Walsh, W. M., & Paulson, S. E. (1994). Families with adolescents: Are we trying to counsel normal behavior? *Family Journal*, 2, 149–157.

Weiner, I. B. (1992). *Psychological disturbance in adolescence* (2d ed.). New York: Wiley.

Wentz, E., Gillberg, I. C., Gillberg, C., & Rastam, M. (2000). Ten-year follow-up of adolescent-onset anorexia nervosa: Physical health and neuro-development. *Developmental Medicine and Child Neurology*, 42, 328–333.

Whiston, S. C., & Sexton, T. L. (1993). An overview of psychotherapy outcome research: Implications for practice. *Professional Psychology: Research and Practice*, 24, 43–51.

Woodside, D. B. (1995). A review of anorexia nervosa and bulimia nervosa. *Current Problems in Pediatrics*, 25, 67–89.

Yalom, I. D. (1995). *The theory and practice of group psychotherapy* (4th ed.). New York: Basic Books.

———, & Lieberman, M. H. (1971). A study of encounter group casualties. *Journal of Abnormal Psychology*, 25, 16–30.

NAME INDEX

SUBJECT INDEX